OVERCOMING
ADDICTIONS

DEEPAK CHOPRA, M.D.

OVERCOMING

ADDICTIONS

the spiritual solution

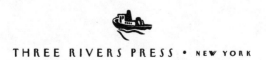

THREE RIVERS PRESS • NEW YORK

Published by Three Rivers Press, New York, New York.
Member of the Crown Publishing Group.

Random House, Inc. New York, Toronto, London, Sydney, Auckland
www.randomhouse.com

THREE RIVERS PRESS is a registered trademark and the Three Rivers Press colophon is a trademark of Random House, Inc.

Printed in the United States of America

Library of Congress Cataloging-in-Publication Data
Chopra, Deepak.
Overcoming addictions : the spiritual solution /
    Deepak Chopra.-1st pbk. ed.
Includes bibliographical references and index.
    1.   Substance abuse-Alternative treatment. 2. Medicine, Ayurvedic.
    I.   Title.
    [RC564.C527 1998]   616.86'06-dc21   97-50046

ISBN 0-609-80195-3

10

CONTENTS

PART ONE

THE MEANING OF ADDICTION

1

THE MISGUIDED SEEKER

I believe that addiction and its consequences are the most serious health problems now facing our society. Cardiovascular disease, respiratory illnesses such as emphysema, many forms of cancer, and AIDS are just a few of the conditions that derive, directly or indirectly, from addiction. This brief book, therefore, is an attempt to address a very large and complex problem in a very limited space. At first glance, this might seem an enormously difficult task. There might even appear to be something presumptuous about trying to deal with the immense complexities of addiction in little more than a hundred pages. Yet I believe that a small book such as this can be of great benefit to the millions of people who are struggling to cope with addictive behaviors in their own lives, and to the millions of family members or loved ones who are trying to help them find a solution to these problems.

In fact, even as I acknowledge the vast scope of our society's difficulties with addiction, I feel very optimistic and eager as I begin this book. The reason is quite simple: although we will be discussing real physical and emotional pain in these pages, essentially this will be a book about health and joy, pleasure and abundance, love and hope.

To some extent, I believe the very positive orientation I will be taking here is unconventional. So much of our effort to address addiction is infused with anger, conflict, and despair. Sometimes this is articulated quite explicitly, as in phrases like "the war on drugs," or in "war stories" of careers ruined and lives shattered by addictive behaviors. At other times the negative orientation expresses itself less directly, as seen in the bleak decor of many treatment centers in which patients are called upon to deal with their problems seated in a circle of plastic chairs in a linoleum-floored, fluorescent-lit room.

Fear of the past, fear of the future, fear of using the present moment for experiencing real joy—so many fears haunt the ways in which we have become immersed in addictive behaviors. Fear is also a part of many treatment programs for addiction. Yet a fear-based approach cannot, in my opinion, be successful for the majority of people over an extended period of time. So I intend to propose here a quite different view of addiction, of what it represents, and of the people who succumb to it.

I see the addict as a seeker, albeit a misguided one. The addict is a person in quest of pleasure, perhaps even of a kind of transcendent experience—and I want to emphasize that this kind of seeking is extremely positive. The addict is looking in the wrong places, but he is going after something very important, and we cannot afford to ignore the meaning of his search. At least initially, the addict hopes to experience something wonderful, something that transcends an unsatisfactory or even an intolerable everyday reality. There's nothing to be ashamed of in this impulse. On the contrary, it provides a foundation for true hope and real transformation.

I'm tempted to go even further in this characterization of the addict as seeker. In my view, a person who has never felt the pull of addictive behavior is someone who has not taken the first faltering step toward discovering the true meaning of Spirit. Perhaps addiction is nothing to be proud of, but it does represent an aspiration toward a higher level of experience. And although that aspiration cannot ultimately be fulfilled by chemicals or by compulsive behaviors, the very attempt suggests the presence of a genuinely spiritual nature.

Ayurveda, the traditional Indian science of health, teaches that there is a memory of perfection within each of us. It is etched into every one of our cells. This memory cannot be erased, but it can be covered over by toxins and impurities of many sorts. Our real task in dealing with addiction lies not so much in pointing out the destructive effects of addictive behaviors but in reawakening the awareness of perfection that always resides within us. As a schoolboy, I read *Paradise Lost,* and it is surely one of the greatest poems in the English language. But I've learned that the paradise within us can never really be lost. We may lose sight of it, yet it is always within our reach.

I've often thought that music is the art form that can best put us in touch with this inner perfection. Although it can certainly be appreciated intellectually and even as a kind of mathematics, music also engages us at a level that's somehow deeper than our conscious thought processes. We can experience this by listening to music, and perhaps even more completely by playing it. Whenever I attend a concert or recital I'm always struck by the obvious effect of the music on the performers. There's a kind of ecstasy being experienced. Musicians who are really caught up in a performance enter a different reality, and they display a totally unself-conscious experience of joy and pleasure. It's a fascinating and inspiring thing to see, and certainly that sort of experience is a worthy aspiration for your own life.

In this connection, I remember reading an account of the life of Charlie Parker, the supremely talented musician who dominated the jazz world in New York City during the 1940s and early 1950s. At their best, his saxophone improvisations were not just stunningly fast and imaginative, they had a coherent logic and unity. The younger musicians who idolized Parker were willing to do anything in order to play the way he could, yet his musical ability seemed almost superhuman. What was the secret of being able to play like that, of being able to enter the privileged space that he so clearly inhabited when he performed?

As it happened, in addition to being a great musician Charlie Parker was also a heroin addict. Although his best solos came when he was off drugs, it became fashionable among a whole generation of jazz musicians to use heroin, and they used it because they were attempting to emulate their idol. The aspiration was understandable and even admirable: they wanted to participate in the kind of transcendent experience they'd seen someone else enjoy. But the results were disastrous for many talented people. For them, heroin proved to be an inadequate, destructive, and false answer to the central purpose of their lives, which was to become great musicians. They hoped to find a shortcut to paradise, but it proved to be a very wrong turn.

This is an absolutely crucial point about addiction, whether it involves drugs, food, alcohol, tobacco, gambling, television soap operas, or any of the thousands of other temptations that every day present themselves in our lives. Addiction begins by looking for the right thing in the wrong place. As the Jungian psychologist Robert Johnson makes clear in his brilliant book *Ecstasy,* addiction is nothing other than a severely degraded substitute for the true experience of joy.

2

NURTURING THE SPIRIT

Man does not live by bread alone.

This well-known metaphor appears in both the Old and New Testaments, and its meaning is not difficult to grasp. Quite simply, it means we have other requirements in life besides the satisfaction of our material needs. But it's important to notice how emphatically this is phrased. Spiritual satisfaction is presented as a fundamental necessity of life, comparable to the need for food. The same point has been made in virtually all other religious and spiritual traditions: we need "food for the soul" in order to survive.

In my opinion, this is quite literally true. The state of our spiritual life has a direct bearing on the functioning of our bodies, including metabolism, digestion, respiration, and all other physiological activities. Yet we have often ignored or misinterpreted our spiritual needs. There is evidence that this is beginning to change, and that a new consciousness of spiritual values is beginning to build, but our long-standing materialistic orientation has had important consequences that are closely connected to the prevalence of addictive behaviors in modern society.

Because we have not sufficiently acknowledged the need for spiritual fulfillment, it should be no surprise that many people have misunderstood the true requirements of the human spirit. They have discovered a wide variety of hyperstimulating activities and an equal number of desensitizing substitutes for the "real thing"—the truly profound experience that Robert Johnson calls *ecstasy*.

This is tragic, because we need ecstasy. We need it in the same basic way that we need food, water, and air, yet this basic human need has been scarcely acknowledged in contemporary Western society. Over the last thirty years we have made great progress in recognizing the deterioration that has been taking place in our physical environment, and in reversing these trends. But at the same time we have failed to acknowledge our spiritual needs with anything like the same fervor. I see the problem of addictive behaviors as a direct result of this fundamental oversight.

In every culture and in every historical epoch, human beings have felt the need for ecstatic experience—for a kind of joy that transcends everyday reality. Various cultures have tried to satisfy this need in many different ways, and some have been much more spiritually oriented than others. In the nineteenth century, the Russian novelist Fyodor Dostoevsky asserted that people need three experiences from their society in order to be content—miracles, mystery, and spiritual guidance—and that these three experiences are much more important to them than the satisfaction of their material needs. Perhaps the addict believes he can gain access to miracles and mystery through his addiction, and this prospect becomes even more enticing in the absence of guidance for the spirit. Rather than seeing addicts as simply weak or even criminal human beings, I choose to see them as people who are responding self-destructively, but still quite understandably, to the spiritual vacuum that exists amid our material abundance.

We all feel the effects of this spiritual vacuum. Depending on who we are and the circumstances in which we find ourselves, we may respond to it in any number of ways. But it's important to recognize that in our society a great many responses to essentially spiritual yearnings take a material form.

I'm reminded of a friend who achieved spectacular success in business while still a young man. In his early forties, he found himself with the means to do or have virtually anything he wanted. And he did want something, too, but he wasn't sure what it really was. In any case, he bought a summer home on a lake. He bought an expensive four-wheel drive vehicle in order to get to the summer home, and in order to have something to do when he got there, he bought a boat. He also bought a state-of-the-art cellular phone, in order to keep track of his business from both his boat and his car. This is a familiar story that has been played out many times by financially successful individuals, and there really is no end to it. After acquiring the home, the car, the boat, and the phone, my friend was really no closer to real fulfillment than he was at the beginning. If anything, he felt somewhat more depressed, and the long-term consequences of this remain to be seen. The boat, for instance, is proving to be a convenient location to do some fairly serious drinking.

Perhaps because my friend is a wealthy person with a fundamentally strong personality, no real harm has so far resulted from his buying spree. But a person with fewer financial resources, or perhaps someone with a different, more vulnerable personality, might find more self-destructive outlets for an unrecognized spiritual craving. Alcohol, drugs, and dangerous sexual behavior are all essentially material responses to a need that is not really physical at its foundation. But if we've never learned where to look for true joy, rather than mere sensation, it's hardly surprising if we don't find it.

In his book, *1939: The Lost World of the Fair,* the computer scientist David Gelernter uses the New York World's Fair as the starting point for an analysis of contemporary society. He draws some conclusions that I find quite clear and convincing. Coming at the end of the Great Depression and just before the outbreak of World War Two, the world's fair offered a vision of the future that at the time must have seemed almost beyond imagining for many people. Someday, the fair suggested, everyone would have a car. What's more, everyone would have a garage to keep it in. There would be affordable homes, electric refrigerators, and even television sets for all. As Gelernter explains, this seemingly impossible vision powered American society through the war years and the period of growing prosperity that followed. And gradually, what had seemed like an unattainable ideal began to be the way many people actually lived. But as success after success was achieved in providing for material needs, there necessarily was a reduction in the number of *things* left to strive for. Since *things* were what we were hoping for and working for, there was a little less hope and a little less purpose as each material goal was achieved.

Today we find ourselves living the dream that inspired us half a century ago. If for many Americans the dream has become an unhappy one, perhaps it's because the dream was constructed for what we needed then. Now that many of us have achieved that, we need something qualitatively different. We need something more.

For the millions of people who have not yet attained the financial and material success that we associate with modern America, the situation is still more complicated. Addictive behavior is surely more prevalent among the poor than among more affluent segments of society, and its effects are all the more destructive among people with diminished social and personal resources. If I tell people who feel excluded from material success that they should acknowledge their spiritual needs, I raise some difficult issues. One might ask, for instance, whether this isn't like telling a small child that being an adult isn't as exciting as it might seem. Children still want to find out for themselves! Yet I do believe that awareness and fulfillment of Spirit is essential to everyone, regardless of their present place in society, and I further believe that this awareness is the only true and permanent answer to addictive behaviors. In the pages that follow, I have tried to show that spiritual fulfillment is available to everyone, regardless of personal history or material resources. Of course, your individual circumstances will certainly influence and illuminate the path you should follow toward developing your spirituality. Indeed, one of the greatest strengths of Ayurveda is its flexibility in serving every individual's unique needs.

I hope that the subtitle of this book emphasizes the depth of my feelings on the subject of addiction. I chose *The Spiritual Solution* because I believe this really is the answer. In chapter 3, I'll discuss in greater detail *why* I believe this to be true, and in subsequent chapters we'll explore *how* you can put *The Spiritual Solution* to work in your own everyday life.

3

ACTION, MEMORY, DESIRE

Whenever I want to understand the meaning of wonder and joy, I think back to a bright and beautiful afternoon when I took a walk with my neighbor's daughter, a little three-year-old girl.

Though our excursion took us only once around the block in a pleasant but unremarkable residential neighborhood, we were gone for almost an hour. Virtually everything we saw or heard was a joyful discovery and the occasion for excited discussion. Again and again we stopped to look at the cars parked along the street. My young friend excitedly discussed their colors, their sizes, their shapes, and she even insisted on touching every single one of them. She devoted the same rapt attention to the flowers growing on the lawns we passed and to the sound of a distant fire engine. When an airplane flew overhead, we immediately stopped and stared at the sky until the plane was just a speck in the distance. And we waved, too, of course.

There were some important things to be learned during that walk around the block. It was clear, for instance, that the little girl's pleasure didn't actually come from any of the things we encountered. The sights and sounds and objects were just opportunities for her to express a feeling that was *already there within her*. The feeling wasn't derived from anything in the external world; instead, it was projected onto the world from her heart and soul. For me, joy is the word that best describes that state of self-generated pleasure.

Most people, or at least most adults, don't experience joy whenever they take a walk around the block, and there are some good reasons for this. Children live in a world of pure contemplation. For them, sights, sounds, and objects exist to be enjoyed or played with, not to be used. But the life of a grown-up is dominated by responsibilities. Walking along on a sunny day, we experience the world around us as a dimly perceived pastiche of colors and textures, while our minds remain focused on whatever problem seems most urgent at the moment. Whatever we may choose to call this level of experience, it clearly is not joy.

But suppose the preoccupied adult, walking along with his eyes on the sidewalk, suddenly finds that something quite unexpected has come into view. It's a hundred-dollar bill! The effect is almost magical! The concerns that seemed so pressing before abruptly vanish, at least for a moment, at this amazing stroke of good fortune. If this were to happen to you, a list of things to do with the hundred-dollar bill would quickly flash before your eyes. Perhaps you wouldn't regard this as a life-transforming experience, but you would almost certainly think of it as something very good—and your state of mind would dramatically change. What would you feel? I'm certain one word instantly comes to mind. You would feel *happiness*.

Finding one hundred dollars makes you happy. The money is an external reason, and happiness is an internal result. Joy, in contrast, might be described as happiness for no reason. Joy is a preexisting internal condition that determines how we experience the world. Joy is a cause, while happiness is an effect.

I'm not suggesting that we, as adults, should always try to experience life as if we were small children, but we should be aware of the joyful state of being that was once ours. It is still always available to us, though it is often confused with the quite different experience that I have called happiness. Happiness is something that we look for, strive for, perhaps even struggle for. Happiness is something that we try to find, or, more likely, something that we try to buy. Joy is something that we are.

People seek to avoid pain and to experience pleasure, and they will take pleasure in whatever form seems available to them. If we've lost touch with our internal sources of joy, if the happiness that originates outside ourselves is the only joy we know, then that is the experience we will seek for ourselves. Depending upon our circumstances, this may be a very positive and fruitful enterprise. Unfortunately, it may also be addiction in one of its many forms.

Let me replace the anecdote about coming across a hundred-dollar bill with some other possibilities. Instead of finding some money, suppose a young man who lives in a world of pain and violence finds a substance that instantly transports him to a completely different experience of life, if only for a short time. Suppose another young man, stalled in his career and feeling the financial pressures of family life, feels more relaxed if he stays up after his wife has gone to bed and drinks a beer—and he feels even better still if he consumes half a dozen of them. For yet another person, this kind of escape might be found somewhere else on the endless list of possibly addictive substances and behaviors. Whatever the experience, if it provides pleasure there will naturally be a desire to repeat it. Repeating it is a choice, at least initially. Later, when addiction has really taken hold, it becomes a need, and even a compulsion.

Ayurveda very clearly identifies the psychological and physiological mechanisms we've been discussing here. Whenever we undertake an action, whether it's picking up a pencil or riding the rapids in a rubber boat, we register that action internally on a spectrum of experience that has great pain at one end and extreme pleasure at the other. Once the action has been completed, it continues to exist in our minds—and in our bodies also—as a memory that is tagged with pain or pleasure of a particular intensity. If the "pain" rating is strong enough, we will do anything in our power to avoid repeating the action. But if the action brought great pleasure, we'll try just as hard to perform that action again.

The Sanskrit word *karma* means action. It can refer to a physical activity or to a mental process such as a thought or an emotion. Every action contains the seeds of memory, which are called *sanskara* in Sanskrit, and the seeds of desire, which are known as *vasana*. The difference between these two concepts is essentially that one looks back while the other looks forward. If the memory of an action is pleasurable, it engenders the desire to perform a new action that will be at least as enjoyable as the original one. Perhaps the new action will simply duplicate what came before, or perhaps it will be an attempt at even greater pleasure.

The essential truth of this paradigm has been recognized even in philosophical traditions far removed from that of India. The French writer Honoré de Balzac observed that in the lives of certain highly emotional people—he referred specifically to gamblers and lovers—there is often a peak experience that comes to dominate all future actions as the individual struggles to re-create the extreme stimulation of that one unique moment. Perhaps without realizing it, Balzac was offering a perfect description of addictive behavior, since gambling and compulsive sex are two of the most well-documented addictions.

Ayurveda emphasizes that once we have performed a specific action it permanently imprints itself on our being, together with its equally enduring components of memory and

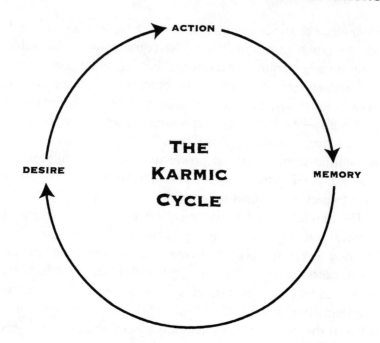

desire. For everything we do or say or even think, an action-memory-desire triad becomes encoded in our cells, and this code simply cannot be erased. This has enormous implications for the approach to addiction that will be offered in this book. We will not try to "get rid of" the memories and desires that underlie addictive behavior. Rather, we will focus on creating new and highly positive feelings that overshadow the destructive impulses of addiction and render them powerless.

Perhaps the best way to illustrate this is through an experience I had with a patient some years ago at our residential treatment center. I believe this case history illustrates the effectiveness of a positive approach to addiction that is designed to suit individual needs. My patient was a seventeen-year-old girl whom I'll call Ellen.

Ellen was having severe health problems when I first saw her, but it quickly became clear that these derived from the drug use and other self-destructive behavior that had domi-

nated her life since she was fourteen. Simply put, Ellen was addicted to heroin, and as a result had become involved in other
dangerous and destructive activities, including theft and pros-
titution.

At first, I decided not to talk with Ellen about any of her addictive behaviors. She had been talking about them with
enough people already. In fact, almost every minute of her life
was focused on addiction in one way or another, either in the
form of participation or of therapeutic intervention. So far,
treatment of any kind had been largely unsuccessful.

"For the moment, let's not discuss any of the problems
you've been having," I suggested to Ellen at one of our first
meetings. "Let's talk about what you did before that. When
you were a young girl, was there anything that you especially
enjoyed doing? What did you really look forward to in those
days? What were you most interested in?"

Ellen thought for a moment, as if she were trying to remember a date from ancient history rather than the events of her
own life just two or three years before. "Well," she said, "I really used to love horseback riding. But I can't even imagine getting on a horse now. I don't even know if I could ride one
without falling off. I was really a different person then."

Looking at Ellen, I could see why she felt that way. She appeared anxious, tired, and underfed. There was a thick layer of
mental, physical, and emotional ill-health insulating her from
the world outside, and even from her own true needs and feelings. So the first goal of her treatment was to remove that bar-
rier. I suggested to Ellen that she take the five-part Ayurvedic
purification procedure known as Panchakarma. After some
discussion, Ellen agreed—and like everyone who experiences
Panchakarma she felt almost "reborn" as a result. Ayurveda
sees mind and body as elements of a single unity. As Ellen's
body was cleansed at the most basic cellular level, her emotions and her spirit were likewise cleansed and restored. There
is nothing mysterious or miraculous about Panchakarma, but

the effect is definitely quite dramatic. The chemical and emotional barriers that had been obscuring Ellen's true self were beginning to be removed.

When she had rested for a few days after these cleansing procedures, I decided it was time to approach the problem of Ellen's addiction more directly. We actually did go horseback riding, despite the misgivings she had expressed earlier. And, as I knew she would, Ellen loved it. From an Ayurvedic perspective, this was tremendously important, because horseback riding rekindled a specific action-memory-desire sequence that had once played a positive part in Ellen's life. I was convinced it could be a positive influence again.

When we returned from the ride, I asked Ellen how she felt. I wanted her to relive the experience she'd just had as she described it to me. Ellen was surprised and pleased that she'd had such a good time in an activity that she'd assumed was no longer available to her. Then I suggested that we go into my office for a moment, where I had something I wanted to discuss with her.

As we sat down on the sofa, I sensed that Ellen was preparing to hear a stern lecture of some kind. I could see that she was silently retreating into the defensive mode that she had used during our early meetings. But instead of talking to Ellen, I once again asked her to talk to me.

"I'd like you to tell me everything you experience when you inject yourself with drugs," I said. "Everything from start to finish. Please describe exactly how it's done, and exactly how it feels."

"You mean what it's like to get high, and then come down?" she asked.

"No, because that's only the end result. Start at the beginning. Tell me how the syringe looks, and how it feels in your hand. Tell me what the needle looks like, and what kind of sensation you feel when you stick it into your arm. If there's pleasure in something, try to describe it to me, and if there's pain or fear or sadness, tell me about that also. Tell me about what you smell when you take drugs, and what kind of sound the syringe makes when you depress the plunger. Is there a particular taste that you experience, or does your mouth feel especially dry? Try to go through the whole event for me in your imagination."

I had several reasons for asking Ellen to do this, but it was most importantly an exercise in *mindfulness*. In Ayurveda, mindfulness means being fully aware of the present moment. It means focusing attention on all your senses and fully experiencing what your body is telling you as you engage in a particular activity. Ellen was not used to being mindful when she injected drugs. It was something that she had learned to do automatically, like a machine, and the fog that quickly enveloped her when the drug took effect even further obscured the actual mechanics of the experience. It was really quite a strain for Ellen, both emotionally and intellectually, to narrate the process for me, but I wanted her to be explicit about what was involved. When she finished with this detailed description, I sensed that the experience had been clearer for her—more real, more mindful—than it would have been if she had actually loaded up a syringe and stuck the needle into her arm, as she had done so many times before.

"Now, just as you've told me in great detail about injecting drugs, I'd like you to tell me again what you experienced when we were out riding those horses this afternoon. Once again, draw upon all your thoughts and all your senses. How did you feel when you first saw the horse today? How did it feel to put your foot in the stirrup? What did the leather of the saddle feel like? How did the horse's hooves sound on the grass? What emotions did you feel at different points in the ride? Take me through the whole thing from beginning to end."

This second description was really much easier for Ellen to provide, and not only because the events had taken place so recently. It was because she had *fully experienced* the horseback ride. Her mind and body were free of the numbness that had overcome her in the past three years. Everything about the horseback ride had been vivid and full of joy for this young girl, and her description of it came across the same way.

"Now you have to choose between those two experiences," I told Ellen, "and since you've just gone through them for me clearly and mindfully, I know you can make an informed decision. Of course, I'm tempted to make a moral comment on the difference between injecting heroin and riding a horse, but I'll resist that temptation, because I don't think it would really have any benefit. I'll just point out that the sights, sounds, scents, textures, thoughts, and feelings you experienced this afternoon will be unavailable to you—literally impossible—if you choose to take drugs."

I'm happy to say that Ellen chose to stay away from drugs, and that she had the strength to follow through on that decision. I believe the approach I took with her involved some risk, but I also believe it was successful for that very reason. I didn't ask Ellen to deny the pleasure she experienced when using heroin. On the contrary, I urged her to sharply focus her attention on those sensations as we talked—but I also asked her to be mindful of the pain associated with drug use. The horseback ride, on the other hand, was pure joy. It was something she had enjoyed before she ever got into trouble, and the reawakened memory of that higher level of pleasure was able to eclipse the relatively low-grade enjoyment of drug use. Once an addict gains access to a deeper form of satisfaction than is possible through self-destructive behavior, the path away from addiction will naturally open up. The memory of inner perfection, once reawakened, creates a desire that is stronger than the addiction itself.

The approach to addiction that worked for Ellen might be called "pleasure based," or perhaps, "mindfulness with an emphasis on pleasure." But it's best just to think of it, quite simply, as *spiritual*. I believe this approach can be successful for a great many people, though the process will sometimes involve some additional steps. Ellen, despite what had happened to her, had the experience of joy to draw upon. Once the positive memories and desires had been held before her, they became powerful forces for her recovery. But suppose Ellen had simply looked at me blankly when I asked her what she had really enjoyed before she became involved with drugs?

There are great numbers of people whose lives have never included the kind of positive moments that Ellen was able to use as healing resources. Or perhaps those moments have been so completely covered over that they can no longer be rekindled by a few pleasant afternoons in the sunshine. You must know the experience of true pleasure before you can renounce the sensations of addictive behaviors. And the first step toward knowing joy is simply knowing yourself. One of Ayurveda's greatest contributions is the way it accommodates the absolute uniqueness of each human being, while at the same time providing categories of mind body types that allow us to understand individual needs and characteristics in a highly practical way.

In the next chapter, you'll have an opportunity to identify your own mind body type within this Ayurvedic system, and later in the book you'll learn how this knowledge can be used to create mental, physical, and spiritual well-being—or, in a single word, *joy*.

4

DISCOVERING YOUR

MIND BODY TYPE

Ayurveda is the world's oldest system for the preservation of health and the prevention and elimination of disease. Its origins date to 2500 B.C., and it had already been in existence for centuries when Hippocrates and the other early Greek physicians did their work. In fact, they were probably influenced by ideas from Indian medicine that had been carried to Europe over well-developed trade routes from the East. Today, as we begin to see the limits of what can be accomplished using a purely mechanistic view of the body, the powerful insights of Ayurveda and other traditional systems of health care are once again assuming major importance in the West.

Perhaps the most important idea in all of Ayurveda is the principle that we must know the patient before we can understand and control the disease. This insight that has been shared by healers in many traditions is sometimes neglected in contemporary health care, where the sheer number of patients and the reliance on widely prescribed drugs can shift the focus away from individual needs. In order really to know the condition of any human being, we must be aware of his or her mental, emotional, and even spiritual makeup as well as height, weight, blood pressure, and all the other physiological signs that modern medicine ordinarily relies upon. Ayurveda teaches that it is even unwise to make a sharp distinction between mind and body: these are simply elements of the single wholeness that comprises any human being. When we are dealing with addiction, the intimate connection between mind and body becomes particularly important. Here the thought or desire for an action is clearly the real source of the problem. The notion of a rigid separation between an emotional state and a physical illness is virtually useless when dealing with addictive behaviors.

Over the centuries, Ayurveda has developed an extremely effective terminology for expressing the connections between mind and body, and for describing the ways in which those connections manifest themselves in any single person. According to Ayurveda, the universe is created, formed, and organized by consciousness, which expresses itself through five great elements: space, air, fire, water, and earth. In the mind body system of a human being, these five elements refine themselves into three essential governing principles that Ayurveda calls *doshas*. It is through the doshas that the energy and information of the universe makes itself present in our bodies and our lives.

Each of the three doshas has a specific influence on the physiology:

Vata dosha is the principle of movement: it governs circulation, the passage of food through the digestive tract, and even the movement of ideas and feelings through our thoughts. Vata is derived from the elements of space and air; like the wind, it is unpredictable and constantly in motion.

Pitta dosha is associated with the element of fire and is often spoken of through metaphors of heat. Pitta is responsible for the conversion of food into energy through the process of digestion, and for the metabolism of air and water as well.

Kapha dosha is the principle of structure in the mind body system. It derives from the elements of earth and water, and is said to be the "heaviest" of the doshas. Kapha is required for the formation of muscle, bone, and sinew; Kapha is even responsible for the cell walls that give structure to your physiology at the most basic level.

Ayurveda teaches that your mind body system is defined by the proportions of Vata, Pitta, and Kapha in your physiology—and by the extent to which the current proportions deviate from your "ideal" doshic balance, which was set at the beginning of your life. If at birth your dominant dosha was Vata, Ayurveda refers to you as a Vata type, because the characteristics of Vata are most evident in your mental and physical makeup. Similarly, if Pitta or Kapha were initially dominant, this means that Pitta or Kapha are most influential in your nature. As your life progresses, however, stress or illness can cause imbalances to occur among the doshas, so that one of the subordinate elements can become dominant. It's also possible for the dominant dosha to go out of balance. An unbalanced Vata type, for instance, could have excessive Vata just as easily as too much Pitta or Kapha.

All three doshas, of course, must be present in your physiology, even in every cell of your body. Because the proportions are constantly shifting as life progresses, a precise determination of your body type and any current imbalance can become fairly complex. That evaluation should best be made in person by a physician trained in Ayurveda. For the purposes of this book, however, you can identify your dominant dosha with the help of the questionnaire that follows. This information can be of great benefit in recognizing your addictive behaviors and the needs and vulnerabilities that underlie them. Please complete the questionnaire now, before you read any further.

AYURVEDA MIND BODY QUESTIONNAIRE

The following quiz is divided into three sections. For the first 20 questions, which apply to Vata dosha, read each statement and mark, from 0 to 6, whether it applies to you.

0 = Doesn't apply to me

3 = Applies to me somewhat (or some of the time)

6 = Applies to me mostly (or nearly all of the time)

At the end of the section, write down your total Vata score. For example, if you mark a 6 for the first question, a 3 for the second, and a 2 for the third, your total up to that point would be 6 + 3 + 2 = 11. Total the entire section in this way, and you will arrive at your final Vata score. Proceed to the 20 questions for Pitta and those for Kapha.

When you are finished, you will have three separate scores. Comparing these will determine your body type.

For fairly objective physical traits, your choice will usually be obvious. For mental traits and behavior, which are more subjective, you should answer according to how you have felt and acted most of your life, or at least for the past few years.

SECTION 1: VATA

	Does not apply		Applies sometimes			Applies most times	
1. I perform activities very quickly.	0	1	2	3	4	5	6
2. I am not good at memorizing things and then remembering them later.	0	1	2	3	4	5	6
3. I am enthusiastic and vivacious by nature.	0	1	2	3	4	5	6
4. I have a thin physique—I don't gain weight very easily.	0	1	2	3	4	5	6
5. I have always learned new things very quickly.	0	1	2	3	4	5	6
6. My characteristic gait while walking is light and quick.	0	1	2	3	4	5	6
7. I tend to have difficulty making decisions.	0	1	2	3	4	5	6

	Does not apply		Applies sometimes		Applies most times	
8. I tend to develop gas and become constipated easily.	0	1	2	3	4	5	6
9. I tend to have cold hands and feet.	0	1	2	3	4	5	6
10. I become anxious or worried frequently.	0	1	2	3	4	5	6
11. I don't tolerate cold weather as well as most people do.	0	1	2	3	4	5	6
12. I speak quickly and my friends think that I'm talkative.	0	1	2	3	4	5	6
13. My moods change easily and I am somewhat emotional by nature.	0	1	2	3	4	5	6
14. I often have difficulty falling asleep or having a sound night's sleep.	0	1	2	3	4	5	6
15. My skin tends to be very dry, especially in winter.	0	1	2	3	4	5	6
16. My mind is very active, sometimes restless, but also very imaginative.	0	1	2	3	4	5	6
17. My movements are quick and active; my energy tends to come in bursts.	0	1	2	3	4	5	6
18. I am easily excitable.	0	1	2	3	4	5	6
19. I tend to be irregular in my eating and sleeping habits.	0	1	2	3	4	5	6
20. I learn quickly, but I also forget quickly.	0	1	2	3	4	5	6

VATA SCORE

SECTION 2: PITTA

	Does not apply		Applies sometimes		Applies most times	
1. I consider myself to be very efficient.	0	1	2	3	4	5	6
2. In my activities, I tend to be extremely precise and orderly.	0	1	2	3	4	5	6

	Does not apply		Applies sometimes			Applies most times	
3. I am strong-minded and have a somewhat forceful manner.	0	1	2	3	4	5	6
4. I feel uncomfortable or become easily fatigued in hot weather— more so than other people.	0	1	2	3	4	5	6
5. I tend to perspire easily.	0	1	2	3	4	5	6
6. Even though I might not always show it, I become irritable or angry quite easily.	0	1	2	3	4	5	6
7. If I skip a meal or a meal is delayed, I become uncomfortable.	0	1	2	3	4	5	6
8. One or more of the following characteristics describes my hair: • early graying or balding • thin, fine, straight • blond, red, or sandy-colored	0	1	2	3	4	5	6
9. I have a strong appetite; if I want to, I can eat quite a large quantity.	0	1	2	3	4	5	6
10. Many people consider me stubborn.	0	1	2	3	4	5	6
11. I am very regular in my bowel habits—it would be more common for me to have loose stools than to be constipated.	0	1	2	3	4	5	6
12. I become impatient very easily.	0	1	2	3	4	5	6
13. I tend to be a perfectionist about details.	0	1	2	3	4	5	6
14. I get angry quite easily, but then I quickly forget about it.	0	1	2	3	4	5	6
15. I am very fond of cold foods, such as ice cream, and also ice-cold drinks.	0	1	2	3	4	5	6
16. I am more likely to feel that a room is too hot than too cold.	0	1	2	3	4	5	6

	Does not apply		Applies sometimes			Applies most times	
17. I don't tolerate foods that are very hot and spicy.	0	1	2	3	4	5	6
18. I am not as tolerant of disagreement as I should be.	0	1	2	3	4	5	6
19. I enjoy challenges, and when I want something I am very determined in my efforts to get it.	0	1	2	3	4	5	6
20. I tend to be quite critical of others and also of myself.	0	1	2	3	4	5	6

PITTA SCORE

SECTION 3: KAPHA

	Does not apply		Applies sometimes			Applies most times	
1. My natural tendency is to do things in a slow and relaxed fashion.	0	1	2	3	4	5	6
2. I gain weight more easily than most people and lose it more slowly.	0	1	2	3	4	5	6
3. I have a placid and calm disposition—I'm not easily ruffled.	0	1	2	3	4	5	6
4. I can skip meals easily without any significant discomfort.	0	1	2	3	4	5	6
5. I have a tendency toward excess mucus or phlegm, chronic congestion, asthma, or sinus problems.	0	1	2	3	4	5	6
6. I must get at least eight hours of sleep in order to be comfortable the next day.	0	1	2	3	4	5	6
7. I sleep very deeply.	0	1	2	3	4	5	6

	Does not apply		Applies sometimes			Applies most times	

8. I am calm by nature and not easily angered.

0 1 2 3 4 5 6

9. I don't learn as quickly as some people, but I have excellent retention and a long memory.

0 1 2 3 4 5 6

10. I have a tendency toward becoming plump—I store extra fat easily.

0 1 2 3 4 5 6

11. Weather that is cool and damp bothers me.

0 1 2 3 4 5 6

12. My hair is thick, dark, and wavy.

0 1 2 3 4 5 6

13. I have smooth, soft skin with a somewhat pale complexion.

0 1 2 3 4 5 6

14. I have a large, solid body build.

0 1 2 3 4 5 6

15. The following words describe me well: serene, sweet-natured, affectionate, and forgiving.

0 1 2 3 4 5 6

16. I have slow digestion, which makes me feel heavy after eating.

0 1 2 3 4 5 6

17. I have very good stamina and physical endurance as well as a steady level of energy.

0 1 2 3 4 5 6

18. I generally walk with a slow, measured gait.

0 1 2 3 4 5 6

19. I have a tendency toward oversleeping and grogginess upon awakening, and am generally slow to get going in the morning.

0 1 2 3 4 5 6

20. I am a slow eater and am slow and methodical in my actions.

0 1 2 3 4 5 6

KAPHA SCORE

FINAL SCORE

VATA   **PITTA**   **KAPHA**

HOW TO DETERMINE YOUR BODY TYPE

Now that you have added up your scores, you can determine your body type. Although there are only three doshas, remember that Ayurveda combines them in ten ways to arrive at ten different body types.

- **If one score is much higher than the others, you are probably a single-dosha type.**
     Single-Dosha Types
     Vata
     Pitta
     Kapha

You are definitely a single-dosha type if your highest score is twice as high as the next highest dosha score (for instance, Vata—90, Pitta—45, Kapha—35). In single-dosha types, the characteristics of Vata, Pitta, or Kapha predominate. Your next highest dosha may still show up in your natural tendencies, but it will be much less distinct.

- **If no single dosha dominates, you are a two-dosha type.**
     Two-Dosha Types
     Vata-Pitta or Pitta-Vata
     Pitta-Kapha or Kapha-Pitta
     Vata-Kapha or Kapha-Vata

If you are a two-dosha type, the traits of your two leading doshas will predominate. The higher one comes first in your body type, but both count.

Most people are two-dosha types. A two-dosha type might have a score like this: Vata—80, Pitta—90, Kapha—20. If this was your score, you would consider yourself to be a Pitta-Vata type.

• If your three scores are nearly equal, you may be a three-dosha type.

    Three-Dosha Type
    Vata-Pitta-Kapha

However, this type is considered rarest of all. Check your answers again, or have a friend go over your responses with you. Also, you can read over the descriptions of Vata, Pitta, and Kapha on pages 31–35 to see if one or two doshas are more prominent in your makeup.

THE THREE DOSHAS AND THEIR CHARACTERISTICS

According to Ayurveda, knowing your body type is the first, all-important step toward genuine good health. This is especially true when dealing with addiction. Although all three doshas must be present in order to sustain life, they are rarely present in equal proportions in any individual, and it's crucial to recognize whether Vata, Pitta, or Kapha is your principle influence. By understanding your dominant dosha, you can learn the areas in which you may become vulnerable when you are under physical or emotional stress—and you can also determine what kinds of activities and changes in your lifestyle can best help you restore balance in mind and body.

VATA

Like a prairie wind, Vata is always in motion, always shifting, always reversing direction. Vata types are much more variable than Pittas or Kaphas, and their behavior from one day to the next is much more difficult to predict. Bursts of energy, both mental and physical, appear suddenly in Vata people, and then vanish just as quickly. Whether walking, or eating, or deciding when to go to sleep, Vatas are consistently inconsistent. This variability is also present in their digestion, their moods and emotions, and the state of their general health. Vatas, for example, are particularly vulnerable to minor illnesses such as colds and flu.

Characteristics of Vata Type

- Light, thin build
- Performs activity quickly
- Irregular hunger and digestion
- Light, interrupted sleep; tendency toward insomnia
- Enthusiasm, vivaciousness, imagination
- Excitability, changing moods
- Quick to grasp new information, also quick to forget
- Tendency to worry
- Tendency to be constipated
- Tires easily, tendency to overexert
- Mental and physical energy comes in bursts

It is very Vata to:

- Be hungry at any time of the day or night
- Love excitement and constant change
- Go to sleep at different times every night, skip meals, and keep irregular habits in general
- Digest food well one day and poorly the next
- Walk quickly
- Display bursts of emotion that are short-lived and quickly forgotten

PITTA

Like a red-hot flame, the defining quality of Pitta is intensity. This association with heat is evident even in the physical characteristics of Pitta types, who often have red hair and florid complexions. By nature, Pittas are ambitious or even driven individuals, with bold styles of self-expression and a tendency to become argumentative if challenged. When in balance, Pitta types are affectionate, and a face glowing with warmth and happiness is characteristic of this dosha. It is only when stress, improper diet, or another destabilizing influence comes into play that the aggressive, critical side of Pitta's nature begins to assert itself.

Characteristics of Pitta Type

- Medium build
- Medium strength and endurance
- Sharp hunger and thirst, strong digestion
- Fair to ruddy skin, often freckled
- Aversion to sun and hot weather
- Enterprising personality, sharp intellect, likes challenges
- Precise, articulate speech
- Cannot skip meals
- Blond, light-brown, or red hair

It is very Pitta to:

- Feel ravenous if dinner is half an hour late
- Live by your watch and resent having your time wasted
- Wake up at night feeling hot and thirsty
- Take command of a situation or feel that you should
- Walk with a determined stride
- Learn from experience that others sometimes find you too demanding or critical

KAPHA

Kapha is the calmest, most stable dosha, and it goes out of balance much less easily than Vata or Pitta. Kapha brings structure and stamina to the physiology, and these characteristics are evident in the stocky builds of many Kapha types. By nature Kaphas are serene and optimistic. They are slow to anger, and prefer to consider all points of view before taking a position of their own. When out of balance, however, Kaphas can become lethargic and indecisive. They benefit from vigorous exercise and a diet that counters their natural tendency toward overweight. Despite these vulnerabilities, Ayurveda describes Kapha people as extremely fortunate: they are naturally loving and considerate, and their innate physical strength provides protection against illness of all kinds.

Characteristics of Kapha Type

- Solid, powerful build; excellent physical strength and endurance
- Steady energy; slow and graceful in action
- Tranquil, relaxed personality; slow to anger
- Cool, smooth, thick, pale, often oily skin
- Slow to grasp new information, but good retentive memory
- Heavy, prolonged sleep
- Tendency toward overweight
- Slow digestion, mild hunger
- Affectionate, tolerant, forgiving
- Tendency to be possessive and complacent

It is very Kapha to:

- Mull things over for a long time before making a decision
- Wake up slowly, lie in bed for a long time, and need coffee upon arising
- Be happy with the status quo and preserve it by conciliating others
- Respect others' feelings, and feel genuine empathy
- Seek emotional comfort from eating

- Have graceful movements and a gliding walk, even if overweight

In Part Two, we'll discuss some of the most common addictive behaviors, paying special attention to the relationship between specific addictions and the doshas. Because unbalanced Vata is responsible for impulsive actions and nervous instability, pacifying this dosha is particularly important in controlling addictive behavior. Unbalanced Pitta is the foundation for the exaggerated sense of self-control that some addicts attribute to themselves, including such beliefs as "I can quit any time I feel like it," or "I can drink as much as I want and it doesn't affect me at all." Kapha types, on the other hand, often really are able to endure more substance abuse than other people. This, combined with Kapha's natural tendency toward inertia and slowness to change, sometimes makes addicted Kapha types challenging to treat.

I strongly urge you to read all the chapters in Part Two, even if you have no personal involvement with a specific addiction. Gaining insight into addictive behaviors that are somewhat different from your own can provide a valuable sense of perspective. It can also help you to understand the feelings of non-addicts—friends, family members, or co-workers—when they are called upon to deal with the complex psychological phenomenon of addiction despite the fact that it may be very far from their own experience.

Part Three provides specific strategies for pacifying the Vata imbalance that is fundamental to all addiction. Once this has been accomplished, balance can be restored to your system as a whole. You can begin to experience the true joy of life, which effortlessly precludes addictive behavior.

While the information in this book can be of great benefit, please be aware that it is not intended as a substitute for professional care in dealing with potentially serious health problems. Addiction originates from a combination of personal, environmental, and societal factors. While I urge you to take responsibility for your own health, I also urge you to be aware of influences that may be beyond your control, or that you may not even be aware of. In any case, please consult your physician before you undertake any new program of diet or exercise such as those described in Part Three. This is especially important when your present condition may be weakened as a result of prolonged addictive behavior.

PART TWO

THE EXPERIENCE
OF ADDICTION

PART TWO

THE EXPERIENCE
TRADITION

5

ALCOHOL ADDICTION

Alcohol, in the form of beer, wine, or hard liquor, serves many purposes in our present society, just as it has since the earliest periods of recorded history. In the Catholic Mass, in the Jewish Passover service, and in the rituals of many other religious faiths, alcohol has a ceremonial, even a sacred function. In the United States we drink champagne to celebrate happy occasions, and countless television commercials remind us that plenty of beer means a good time will be had by all. This is the outgrowth of a long tradition in the West. Describing the importance of alcohol in the social life of seventeenth-century England, one historian has written that drink was "built into the fabric of social life. It played a part in nearly every public and private ceremony, every commercial bargain, every craft ritual, every private occasion of mourning or rejoicing."

Side by side with the central role of alcohol, however, there exists a long tradition of hostility to drinking. In America this hostility reached a high point during the Prohibition period of the 1920s and early 1930s. Even without Prohibition, however, the use of alcohol in the American population as a whole has been generally falling over the years, after reaching a peak roughly 150 years ago. In 1830, the estimated per capita consumption of pure alcohol was 7.1 gallons per year, while in 1989 the figure was only 2.43 gallons.

Even the 1989 figure, however, translates to 576 cans of beer for every American, so it's clear that a great deal of drinking is still taking place. But the majority of it is being done by a relatively small number of people: studies have shown that 50 percent of all alcoholic beverages are consumed by only 10 percent of the total number of drinkers. This 10 percent comprises the group of alcoholic and alcohol-dependent individuals to whom this chapter is principally addressed.

THE BENEFITS OF ALCOHOL

As we discussed in connection with my young patient Ellen and her drug addiction, I believe it's essential to acknowledge the pleasures of addictive substances as well as their destructive effects. Certainly many pleasures are associated with alcohol use, and there are even documented health benefits. Of course, once "use" becomes "abuse," the positive effects are greatly outweighed by the dangers, as will certainly become clear.

One may wonder how humans began drinking alcohol in the first place. Historians believe that early man may have seen animals eating fermented fruits and noticed the dramatic effects on their behavior. Some adventurous individuals must have decided to find out exactly what was making that deer stagger around. From there, it was probably not long before people were producing alcoholic beverages as a highly developed skill, or even an art.

For many thousands of years, alcoholic beverages and the

techniques needed to produce them have been woven into the fabric of human civilization. The recent discovery in Iran of a jar containing residues of alcohol indicates that wine was being produced in the Middle East more than seven thousand years ago. One historian has observed that there are only two universal innovations that are shared by all cultures. The first of these universals is the development of some form of bread or pasta, and the second is the "discovery and use of the natural fermentation process." Wine, of course, is frequently mentioned in the Bible, with both positive and negative connotations. The ancient Greek historian Herodotus reports that the rulers of the Persian empire would not arrive at a final decision on any important matter until they had discussed it both sober and drunk. And one of Plato's most beautiful and important dialogues, the discussion of love entitled *The Symposium*, records the uninhibited conversation at a drinking party; literally translated, the Greek word *symposium* means "to drink together." Drinking is also frequently mentioned (and celebrated) by Shakespeare, and it has had an important place in the work of innumerable other writers and artists—to say nothing of what it has meant in their own lives.

Along with the historical importance of alcohol itself, drinking has been the basis for social institutions that continue to be important today. The television show *Cheers* offers the vision of a neighborhood tavern as a kind of paradise: a warm setting where a group of long-standing friends meet, talk, and get into humorous complications. The show rarely ventures away from the tavern location, and in fact doing so would undermine the whole meaning of the program. The tavern can be a refuge, a safe place in which to get away, as the title of the short story by Ernest Hemingway about a Spanish café suggests: "A Clean, Well-Lighted Place."

Gathering places organized around social drinking can undoubtedly provide emotional benefits, and any genuine experience of happiness or relaxation has physiological benefits as well. Furthermore, the medical as well as the popular view of alcohol has been altered somewhat by studies showing that moderate drinking can reduce the risk of heart attacks. Although this benefit has been associated with changes in blood chemistry, it may derive as much from lowered stress levels as from any biochemical effects.

Since prehistoric times, alcohol has played a varied but extremely important part in human experience. On the one hand, it has been used in sacraments and religious ceremonies as a way of getting in touch with the gods. On the other, alcohol has helped people feel closer to one another. In its dual role as both sacred and profane, alcohol could be compared with fire as a structural principle in our lives. And, again like fire, it can easily get out of control.

THE DANGERS OF ALCOHOL

Alcoholic beverages can be thought of as drinks, but they can also be defined as drugs. In fact, alcohol is by far the most abused drug in the United States. One important study proposes that alcohol accounts for 85 percent of America's total drug addiction problem. In addition, there is evidence that approximately 13.5 percent of the total population will meet the diagnostic criteria for alcohol addiction or dependence at some point in their lives.

The consequences of these statistics are extremely serious for both the individual and for society. Certain forms of cancer, for example, are specifically associated with heavy drinking, and as much as 75 percent of all deaths from cancer of the esophagus are related to alcohol use. Cancer of the liver is also a frequent complication of the general destruction of that organ brought about by excessive alcohol intake. Damage to the pancreas, stomach, and small intestine can also result from prolonged heavy drinking, as can deterioration of mental functioning. Indeed, a detailed list of the devastation wrought upon the body by alcohol abuse could go on for many pages, as could a tally of treatment cost.

The dangers of alcohol are not limited to its biochemical effects. Although significant progress has been made in recent years, the high correlation between drinking and automobile accidents is well-known; approximately half of all motor vehicle deaths are still alcohol related. Sixty percent of all boating fatalities involve alcohol. In addition, approximately 30,000 people are killed each year as a result of non-motor-vehicle-related accidents of various types. It's important to note that these accident figures do not refer just to victims who were heavily intoxicated. Virtually any use of alcohol dramatically raises the chances of accidental injury.

The problems caused by alcohol abuse are extremely significant at a less dire level as well. Drinking is a frequent cause of insomnia, for example. Obesity can also be associated with alcohol, as can a form of anorexia prevalent among heavy drinkers, some of whom eat almost nothing and derive their entire daily caloric intake from alcohol. Hangovers can also be quite unpleasant, and despite the many folk remedies for the problem, the precise biological mechanism of a hangover is still not well understood.

Again, this is only a brief glimpse into the inferno of punishments that await the heavy user of alcohol. It's important, however, to look more closely at what constitutes "heavy" use and at the distinctions that have been drawn between alcohol dependency and truly addictive behavior.

ALCOHOL DEPENDENCE AND ALCOHOL ADDICTION

As a physician trained in Ayurveda, I am uneasy with the idea that a well-defined line exists between the physical and the mental, emotional, and spiritual elements of our nature. Since every thought and feeling has physical manifestations throughout our physiology, it's clear that the mind and the body are truly one. Nevertheless, perhaps a useful distinction can be made between alcohol dependence and addiction by separating experiences that are perceived as primarily emotional from those that give rise to well-defined physical sensations. In addition, the term alcohol addiction can be distinguished from alcohol dependence by the presence of serious, clearly defined negative elements in the drinker's life, including work disturbances, legal and financial troubles, and family problems that may often include violence. Alcohol dependence, on the other hand, is a more diffuse category in which drinking impedes or intrudes *in any way* upon a person's freedom to enjoy life, however insignificant this interference may seem.

I once was traveling with a friend who enjoyed wine with his meals, as do millions of people all over the world. When we inadvertently found ourselves in a restaurant that did not have a license to sell liquor, however, I came to see that my friend didn't simply enjoy wine with dinner; rather, he couldn't enjoy dinner without wine. When we realized that the restaurant couldn't provide any, eating there was simply out of the question because of the genuine misery that this imposed on my friend. "I just can't eat without wine," he sadly apologized, as we looked for another restaurant. He had an inflexible, consistent need for alcohol at certain times of the day. If alcohol was not present at his mealtimes, my friend became intensely uncomfortable and needed to remedy the situation. Unlike a fully developed alcoholic, however, he did not become physically ill when liquor was withdrawn, nor were the outward circumstances of his life noticeably affected. Although alcohol played only a small and specific role in his life, he was dependent according to my understanding of the term.

In contrast to dependence, fully developed alcoholism—that is, alcohol addiction—can be defined more specifically than alcohol dependence, and it can be identified through a limited number of well-documented traits and characteristics.

- *Prioritizing.* Drinking is a primary focus of the alcoholic's day. Important activities are rescheduled or sacrificed to facilitate drinking, despite any difficulties this may cause. Similarly, an alcoholic recognizes certain times of the day when drinking simply must occur, and he or she makes whatever adjustments are necessary to ensure that this is possible.
- *Increased Tolerance.* Over time, greater amounts of alcohol are needed to bring about the hoped-for effects.
- *Withdrawal Symptoms.* As tolerance of alcohol increases, the unpleasant or even painful symptoms of alcohol withdrawal also increase. These symptoms include shaking, insomnia, agitation, anxiety, and confusion. Eventually this evolves into a vicious circle, and avoidance of these symptoms becomes a major motivator for alcohol use. The alcoholic drinks more in order to avoid the consequences of not drinking, but increased drinking only makes the consequences worse.
- *Craving.* There is often an overwhelming desire or need for a drink, especially when an attempt is being made to reduce drinking. Even with a drink in his or her hand, an alcoholic may already feel the need for the next drink. In a bar or tavern, an alcoholic may actually order a second drink before finishing the first one.
- *Internal Conflict.* As drinking becomes more serious and begins to get out of control, there will be periods in which an alcoholic feels a desire to quit, and he or she may in fact do so for a period of time. When drinking resumes, however, the alcoholic quickly falls back into familiar, well-developed patterns.

• *External Problems.* Difficulties at work, with friends and
family, and with the police are almost certain to occur in an alcoholic's life. In order to avoid these problems, he or she may
become more secretive about drinking, and may hide bottles at
home or at work.

FROM DEPENDENCY TO ADDICTION

It isn't surprising that alcohol dependency frequently develops
into full-blown alcohol addiction. This progression was described in great detail in a series of lectures presented at Yale
University by the researcher E. M. Jellinek. These lectures were
derived from questionnaires completed by more than two
thousand alcoholics, and they are the basis for the "disease
model" of alcoholism, currently an extremely influential approach to treating this problem. As a result of his research,
Jellinek was able to identify specific and predictable stages of
the alcoholic's "disease," although many months or even years
may elapse between the appearance of the various stages.
Alcoholism, in this view, can be understood as a chronic, sys-
temic, degenerative health problem, analogous to incapacitat-
ing diseases such as syphilis or multiple sclerosis. Although
Jellinek recognized that certain drinkers never advance beyond
a "habitual" stage resembling alcohol dependency, he con-
cluded that alcohol addiction progresses through four succinct
stages.

THE DISEASE MODEL OF ALCOHOLISM

First Stage

When using alcohol, the subject experiences dramatically
reduced stress and lowered levels of tension. Over a period of
six months to two years, the future alcoholic begins to drink

almost every day in order to achieve this experience of relaxation. Typically, he or she has a higher tolerance for alcohol than the average person.

Second Stage

When blackouts or memory losses suddenly begin to appear, the second stage of alcoholism has been reached. The blackouts usually involve intermediate memory, such as activities or conversations that took place during a period of drinking on the previous day. Memories of events both before and after the blackout remain unaffected. During this stage, the subject begins to realize that his or her drinking has reached a new level, and tension or guilt becomes associated with the activity. Drinking may begin to take place in secret.

Third Stage

In Jellinek's original formulation, this is the crucial phase in which the drinker moves from more or less controlled intention to out-of-control behavior. The addict now immediately and reflexively responds to tension by drinking, and may even cause or fabricate incidents to justify drinking. Often, the addict begins each day with a drink, and spends the evening becoming seriously intoxicated. This stage may continue for many years, during which the addict remains able to hold a job and function socially, although close relationships become deeply strained.

Fourth Stage

Jellinek referred to this as the chronic phase of alcohol addiction, and it is marked by prolonged periods of intoxication. There are serious problems involving physical and mental health, personal and professional relationships, and the police. Even brief withdrawal from alcohol produces unpleasant and frightening symptoms, and the addict drinks in order to avoid them. Tolerance for alcohol abruptly diminishes, and even small amounts of liquor now cause drunkenness.

During the fourth stage of Jellinek's disease model, a small majority of alcoholics (about 60 percent) undergo an experience that has important implications for the successful treatment of alcoholism. As these people "hit bottom" and feel themselves caught up in total despair, they quite unexpectedly experience a new spiritual awareness. They begin to call upon a higher power to lift them out of the depths to which they have sunk. A small percentage of alcoholics even experience a moment of dramatic revelation, similar to a religious conversion, in which they recognize that they are in the hands of some supreme destiny. In other words, they experience a sort of ecstasy.

This transcendent phenomenon is as equally well documented as the other stages of the alcoholic disease. Perhaps the disease itself could even be interpreted as a deluded attempt to reach this point—a descent into hell that must precede the vision of paradise. In this connection, it may be useful to recall our discussion in chapter 1 of the addict as a misguided seeker, and to quote a letter from the psychologist Carl Jung in which he explicitly creates an analogy between addiction and hell:

> I am strongly convinced that the evil principle prevailing in the world leads the unrecognized spiritual need into perdition, if it is not counteracted either by real religious insight or by the protective wall of human community. An ordinary man, not protected by an action from above and isolated in society, cannot

> *resist the power of evil, which is called very aptly the Devil. . . . "Alcohol" in Latin is "spiritus," the same word for the highest religious experience as well as for the most depraving poison.*

If the pun doesn't seem too far-fetched, one might observe that for a significant number of people the "spiritual solution" of alcohol eventually leads to a spiritual solution for alcoholism. The philosopher William James, in *The Varieties of Religious Experience,* wrote that the real cure for excessive drinking is passionate religion. I am tempted to go even further by saying that the *only* cure for addiction of any sort is the discovery of an intensely felt inner spirituality. Then, upon this spiritual foundation, the recovering addict can begin making the practical changes in his or her life that are necessary for real transformation.

THE MIRACLE OR THE MACHINE?

A quick look at some of the many treatment alternatives for alcoholism may help to clarify my belief in a spiritually based approach. The antithesis of this approach, for example, can be found in the use of alcohol-antagonistic drugs, of which Antabuse is the most common. By blocking the body's ability to metabolize alcohol normally, Antabuse causes a rapid buildup of toxins when a drink is ingested. Violent nausea, headache, a sudden drop in blood pressure, and intense fear of death occur very quickly. In behaviorist terms, the drug provides strong and immediate negative reinforcement for drinking—punishment, in other words. The effects of the drug can even be fatal, and as the addict knows this, there should be a strong disincentive to drink.

For certain individuals, the fear on which Antabuse depends can be effective. Since the drug stays in the system for up to seventy-two hours after the last dose was taken, an addict who feels a sudden impulse to drink will at least give it a second thought before opening the bottle, even if he or she stopped taking the drug several days before. But the impulse to drink has not really been addressed, nor has the memory of inner perfection been reawakened. Rather, the chemical approach to the pain felt by a struggling alcoholic simply threatens an even greater pain if his or her struggle is unsuccessful.

Pain of a different sort underlies many interpersonal, confrontational approaches to treating alcoholism. Here a therapist and/or other addicts in treatment may aggressively inform the subject of the damage caused by his or her drinking and of the self-deluding nature of the alcoholic's thoughts and actions. Elements of this approach play a part in many residential treatment programs for alcoholism, and to some extent in Alcoholics Anonymous as well. As with Antabuse, there can be benefits from confrontation; from an Ayurvedic point of view, it would seem to be most attractive to Pitta types, who are likely to assert their total mastery of a situation no matter how badly it has gotten out of hand. Yet the experience of confrontation can further irritate an already unbalanced Pitta constitution, and may do considerably more harm than good. Ultimately, confrontation is just as likely to raise an addict's defenses as to lower them, and studies have indicated that heightened levels of confrontation also bring about heightened levels of resistance.

Supportive, insight-oriented therapy, which is widely applied not only for substance abuse but for emotional problems of all forms, is based on the idea that an alcoholic's drinking derives from an inner conflict that will diminish as it becomes better understood. Alcoholism is seen as a symptom of an underlying problem within the psyche of the alcoholic. To some extent, the truth of this seems obvious and beyond dispute. But as Arnold Ludwig, M.D., makes clear in his book *Understand-*

ing the Alcoholic's Mind, there are also limits to the effectiveness of insight therapy, whether conducted individually or in groups.

To illustrate these limits, Ludwig introduces the term "state-dependent learning." This refers to the fact that our grasp of an idea, or even our experience of a powerful inner revelation, may not be transferable to all the many settings in which we are likely to find ourselves. This is especially true for a strongly addictive habit such as alcoholism, which can thoroughly dominate an individual's daily life, except perhaps during therapy sessions.

When a group of alcoholics are sitting around a table in the company of a trained therapist, important information can emerge, providing deep understanding of past and present influences on behavior. A self-reflective mood is created in which people are eager to learn and change. This is a unique environment, both physically and emotionally, and a very different environment from a bar or a restaurant or a home life in which fatigue or stress can trigger the urge to drink. Moreover, once he begins drinking, an alcoholic may become a very different person from what he was during a therapy session. He may literally be unable to remember the session, just as he may later be unable to remember what he said or did while drinking. This kind of amnesia can even exist between various levels of intoxication, and in his book Dr. Ludwig ironically suggests the possibility of insight-oriented therapy sessions while clients are getting drunk. This is not intended as a realistic option, but it does dramatize the problem an alcoholic faces in trying to transfer therapeutic benefits from one setting to another.

Drinking's power to transform an addict into a different person is addressed directly by Alcoholics Anonymous, and this organization certainly represents one of the most powerful approaches to alcoholism ever developed. By emphasizing avoidance of the first drink, AA urges the addict to prevent the destructive effects of alcohol from ever getting started. This is necessary because for an addict the destructive effects are in some sense always present—he or she is always an alcoholic, with all the vulnerability that implies, regardless of whether any drinking actually takes place. As the first of AA's famous Twelve Steps makes clear, the addict must understand that he or she is *powerless* over alcohol—and that once a drink is taken, a long-standing member of AA has no more sobriety than a drinker who has never even heard of the organization.

Many books have been written about Alcoholics Anonymous, including both scientific evaluations and personal narratives. I urge anyone who is concerned with the problem of alcoholism to learn more about this organization, either by reading or by attending an open meeting of an AA group. For our purposes here, and without going into great detail, I would like to point out what I see as the benefits of AA's approach, as well as what appear to me to be shortcomings.

A great strength of Alcoholics Anonymous, and the other twelve-step programs it has inspired, is their recognition of a higher spiritual power that must be called upon if the problem of addiction is to be solved. In addition, the purely voluntary nature of the organization—and the absence of a hierarchical structure or any authoritarian presence—allows the addict to assume full responsibility for recovery.

But I believe the most remarkable aspect of AA is the fact that only the first of the twelve steps makes any mention of alcohol. This has at least two very important effects. First, it makes the point that addictive drinking is not simply a matter of what is in the glass but of what is in the mind and heart as well. Furthermore, it offers the recovering alcoholic a chance to understand drinking not only as an affliction, but as a kind of opportunity, the first rung on a ladder of self-development that can lead to genuine spiritual fulfillment. The Twelve Steps of Alcoholics Anonymous are not just a program for becoming a sober person. They are about becoming a truly *great* person in all areas of life.

Much as I admire these aspects of AA, I am less comfortable with what seems to be a fear-based element in the recovery program. Certainly many alcoholics have developed self-deluding ego mechanisms that need to be broken down, but AA's emphasis on the powerlessness of the addict seems troubling. As he walks a tightrope between the evil strength of alcohol on one side and the saving grace of a higher spiritual power on the other, the addict's true inner nature remains unknown and perhaps even irrelevant. Quite simply, he is what he does—and he himself can never be sure what he's going to do from one day to the next. As AA's best-known maxim puts it, "One day at a time."

From an Ayurvedic perspective, the essence of human nature is not so indeterminate. As children, we all had laughter in our hearts and found joy all around us. That happy child is still within us, in every cell of our beings, and the natural impulse toward health and happiness is always present. We are not emotionally or spiritually neutral, nor are we equally inclined to do harm to ourselves as to do good. Our true, inborn orientation is toward what is good for us and away from what is harmful. There is no real need, therefore, for an attitude of constant vigilance against the dangers of alcohol, or anything else. These dangers and temptations will vanish like mist when our enjoyment of life's real pleasures once again becomes available.

ALCOHOLISM AND THE DOSHAS

Alcoholism and Vata

Prolonged addictive behavior almost always results in a serious Vata imbalance, and this can become even more acute under the stresses of withdrawal from alcohol. Relaxation techniques that balance Vata, therefore, should be given first priority in recovery from alcohol addiction, even if Vata is not normally your dominant dosha.

If you answer yes to two or more of the questions below, you are very likely experiencing a Vata imbalance associated with alcoholism.

1. Do you often feel that your thoughts are restless and scattered, and do you drink in order to feel calmer and more focused?
2. Do you often experience insomnia, and do you drink in order to fall asleep?
3. Do your hands or head sometimes tremble uncontrollably?
4. Have you experienced a noticeable loss of appetite, when you would rather drink than eat?
5. Have you noticed sudden losses of memory or concentration?
6. Do you sometimes feel apathetic about life in general, with an absence of all desire?
7. Are you easily startled or frightened, and do you drink to lessen this?
8. Do even familiar settings sometimes look distant and unreal to you, especially when you drink?
9. Have you ever fainted during or after drinking?
10. Have you ever experienced delusions or hallucinations during or after drinking?

Alcoholism and Pitta

In his authoritative book entitled *Ayurvedic Healing,* Dr. David Frawley emphasizes the fact that alcohol adds sudden and often excessive heat to the body. This aggravates Pitta and can cause inflammatory disorders in the liver and other areas of the digestive system, particularly in Pitta-dominant individuals.

Pitta-dominant people often display characteristic behaviors involving alcohol, and these strong-willed individuals can be very resistant to change. In fact, even seriously alcoholic Pittas frequently deny the existence of any problem whatsoever. They deny it not only to others, but to themselves as well. If your results on the mind body questionnaire indicate that Pitta is your dominant dosha, and if you sometimes suspect that you might be drinking to excess, read the ten questions below. Answering yes to more than two of them is strong evidence that you may be an alcoholic Pitta.

1. Do you wait until a certain time of day to start drinking, and does this seem to you to be proof of your self-control?

2. Do you find yourself looking forward to your "cocktail hour"?

3. Do you ritualize aspects of your drinking, by demanding certain ingredients, mixtures, types of glasses, etc.?

4. Do you ever stop drinking for a few days or weeks to prove you can do it?

5. When drinking, do you sometimes feel like you're competing against other drinkers—or against the alcohol itself—to show how much you can take?

6. When drinking, do you feel contempt for people who act drunk or tipsy?

7. Do you ever combine alcohol with athletics, as in pickup softball or basketball games, or when playing golf?

8. When drinking with others, do you find yourself keeping track of who is buying and when it's your turn to buy a round?

9. Do you become angry and argumentative when you drink?

10. Do you feel that your daily life is a struggle, for which drinking is a respite or a reward?

Alcoholism and Kapha

Nutritionally, alcohol is a form of sugar, and many cases of alcoholism may be manifestations of sugar addiction. This is most frequent among Kapha types, who often have an innate fondness for sugar in any form. Kaphas are especially susceptible to the "yo-yo effect" that accompanies the ingestion of sugar in large amounts, whether in the form of alcohol, candy, or any other sweet. After a brief "high," a sense of physical weakness or lethargy and emotional depression comes on strongly. Since Kaphas are vulnerable to depression in any case, this sequence is very pronounced in unbalanced Kapha types. A deeply alcoholic Kapha is likely to be a severely depressed individual, prone to excessive sleep, obesity, solitary drinking, and even thoughts of suicide.

If you answer yes to two or more of the following questions, this is strong evidence that you are an alcoholic Kapha type.

1. Are you seriously overweight, and do you notice that your drinking has made this worse?
2. Do you often drink alone in your home?
3. Do you sometimes drink in bed?
4. After drinking, do you often sleep for long periods?
5. Do you like alcoholic drinks that include sugar, or that are mixed with soft drinks?
6. Do you notice that you're naturally able to drink more than other people?
7. When drinking, do you initially feel giddy or jolly?
8. After drinking for a while, do you often begin to feel sad or sentimental?
9. Do you sometimes perspire heavily while drinking?

10. After drinking at night, do you often notice congestion in your throat or chest the next morning?

If your answers to these questions indicate the presence of a drinking problem, the Ayurvedic techniques presented in Part Three can help you begin to deal with this. Once again, however, it's wise to have a professional medical evaluation if you suspect you may be an alcoholic.

6

ADDICTION TO

ILLEGAL DRUGS

The dream of a substance that transforms reality is deeply rooted in the human imagination. Vedic literature contains many references to a mystical liquid called soma, the nectar of the gods, which confers immortality on anyone who tastes it, and in Greek mythology ambrosia is said to have the same power. In the Book of Exodus in the Old Testament, the Israelites faced starvation in the desert until God provided manna, a substance that fell like snow from the sky and that tasted like any food that could be imagined.

The Bible contains several ideas that can help us understand the nature of addiction, particularly addiction to drugs. Drug addiction takes hold among men and women whose daily life is like wandering through a desert, bereft of all pleasure and spiritual nourishment. When something offers to transport such people to an entirely different reality, many of them accept the offer simply because nothing else seems to promise anything at all. But as we saw with alcohol, it's one of the ironies of addiction that what begins as a search for pleasure soon evolves into a constant struggle to avoid pain. In most advanced drug addictions, the debilitating effects of withdrawal loom larger than the pleasures of any euphoric high—and the high becomes almost impossible to attain in any case, as the body develops a tolerance to the addictive substance. Soon the drug habit exists simply to keep withdrawal symptoms at bay, and it becomes clear that what may have seemed like the gates of paradise have simply opened on just another desert after all.

The view of addiction as a futile but understandable search runs counter to aspects of the disease theory of addictive behavior that is the foundation of many treatment programs. This theory emphasizes genetic predisposition to the "infection" of addictive behavior, which, once established, acts upon the victim in much the same way as any other infectious disease. Some proponents of this view assert that just one experience of an addictive drug causes a permanent change in the brain chemistry of the user, which gives rise to an equally permanent craving for more drugs. Exposure to drugs is comparable to being bitten by a mosquito carrying malaria or yellow fever. As soon as it starts, the course is set and the damage is done.

But there are some fairly obvious differences between the progress of addiction and the course of an infectious disease. Once bitten by a disease-carrying mosquito, a victim does not need to participate consciously for the infection to take hold. A whole series of more or less voluntary actions, however, must be undertaken by a drug user, and at each point "escape" exists, at least as a physical possibility. The addict must find a supplier, pay for drugs, and often complete a complex sequence of preparations before the drugs can actually be used. The addict must also choose to engage in an activity that is emphatically stigmatized both legally and morally by society at large, and that carries the possibility of severe penalties. All these steps require choices. I prefer to think they are conscious choices, because this opens the possibility that different decisions can be made in their place.

Choice, in my opinion, is really the foundation of healing. These choices must take place at every level of an individual's existence, from the conscious thoughts that direct behavior in the larger world to the biochemical choices made by millions of cells throughout the body. As the psychoanalyst Thomas Szasz has pointed out, societies throughout history have found many different ways to condemn so-called deviant behaviors. Most often this condemnation was on religious grounds, though enforcement of religious orthodoxy was frequently a mask for political power and control. Today our belief in science leads us toward a different terminology of disapproval, and drug use is seen as sick rather than as blasphemous. I believe we must use the disease model of addiction with great caution, and we must always remember that the power to cure always resides within the patient, and not in a particular doctor, treatment facility, or medication. The real task of a physician is to create conditions in which the patient's natural healing powers are able to operate effectively—that is, conditions in which the patient's body and spirit can make the natural choice of health rather than illness, and of joy rather than pain.

As this book is being written, a new campaign against heroin use is being introduced by the Partnership for a Drug-Free America, a nonprofit alliance of media and advertising companies that has created and sponsored anti-drug messages for a number of years. The newly announced messages will appear both in print and on television. They include testimonies from former heroin addicts, as well as ironic juxtapositions of the drug's effects with the glamorous image it may hold for prospective users. A media campaign such as this raises important questions. To the extent that it portrays drug use as a misguided strategy for achieving pleasure or personal power, I believe it is on target. But a focus on the ravages of drug use is likely to be ineffective, just as the probability of eventually getting arrested has little effect on most individuals who commit crimes. People who use heroin in this society are not particularly vulnerable to fear of what might happen to them. They're frightened and depressed about what has already happened to them, although they may not be fully conscious of that fact. The sources of real joy in their lives are so diminished that the superficial pleasures of heroin and other drugs loom large by comparison. Even before they touch heroin for the first time, these people are profoundly suffering. What they need is joy in the fullest sense of the word. They already know quite enough about pain.

DEFINING POINTS OF DRUG ADDICTION

From an Ayurvedic viewpoint, the absence of joy from one's life is the most important cause as well as the fundamental effect of addiction. But there are also certain clearly recognizable signs of habitual drug use that are evident in an addict's everyday life. These are worthy of attention both diagnostically and for what they reveal about the psychology of an addicted person.

The list of potentially addictive drugs is very long, and there are many distinctions to be made among the biological, psychological, and social characteristics of the various substances. Cocaine in its powdered form, for example, is a middle- or upper-class drug as a rule, and its effect on the body differs from rock cocaine, or crack, which is sold in lower-priced units and is more popular among economically depressed populations. Amphetamines are often used by both long-distance truck drivers and university students, while the use of opiates such as heroin is present to some extent in virtually all segments of the population. But despite the differences among the various drugs and the people who use them, certain defining elements are common to addiction in general. Instead of considering each drug individually, therefore, or by pharmacological class, we will focus in this section on the shared hallmarks of addictive behavior as a whole.

As with alcohol, the use of drugs for mind-altering or

"recreational" purposes has been a part of human culture—
every human culture—for many thousands of years. Analysis
of clay tablets created almost seven thousand years ago, in the
Middle Eastern kingdom of Sumeria, reveals a hieroglyphic
word for opium, and the context suggests that this word had
connotations of joy and rejoicing. There is also evidence that
the Lake Dwellers of Switzerland, whose culture dates from
around 2500 B.C., ate poppy seeds, which are the natural
source of opium and opium derivatives, such as heroin and
morphine. By asserting that drug use has existed since the
dawn of recorded history, however, I do not mean to condone
it. Indeed, the impulse of human society to stigmatize or pro-
hibit certain behaviors is every bit as ancient as the desire to
use drugs or alcohol. One of its earliest expressions occurs in
the biblical story of Adam and Eve, who violated God's prohibition by eating fruit from the Tree of Knowledge. We cannot,
therefore, defend drug use simply on the basis that it's something quite "natural" for human beings, because it's also natural for them to label some actions as good and others as bad.
Quite often these labels have been applied arbitrarily, however,
and what was good in one century has often turned into bad in
another. So to discuss drug use intelligently and objectively, we
will need to consider social and historical variables as well as
medical and psychological factors.

Coffee, for example, is not presently considered an illicit
drug in contemporary Western society, despite the fact that
heavy coffee use can cause both physical and emotional problems. When it first appeared in Europe in the seventeenth century, coffee at once became extremely popular, and efforts
were made by the civil authorities to regulate or even outlaw
its use. This proved impossible, however, and coffeehouses became popular gathering places all across the continent.
Voltaire and other important figures of the Enlightenment
were coffee lovers, and the French novelist Balzac literally died
of his coffee addiction, which was so pronounced that he even-

tually consumed his coffee in the form of a thick soup. Today coffee dependence and even addiction is common in the United States and Europe, and we can see clearly defined withdrawal symptoms among coffee drinkers who are abruptly denied access to the beverage. But we think of coffee as a drink, not as a drug. Similarly, heavy consumers of chocolate and sugar meet many of the criteria for drug addiction, but we intuitively place them in a different category than users of heroin or cocaine.

The fact that certain drugs are illegal is probably a fundamental part of their allure. By choosing to use these substances, an individual rejects and separates from the values of mainstream society and joins a subgroup whose lives are defined by addiction. This is a basic element in the psychology of drug use. If heroin or cocaine were legalized tomorrow, which I do not advocate, I believe that most addicts would still find reasons for obtaining these drugs illegally, as well as ways to do so.

The present criteria for drug addiction are clearly defined in the *Diagnostic and Statistical Manual of Mental Disorders, Fourth Edition* (1994), published by the American Psychiatric Association, and it will be useful to discuss briefly each of these criteria individually before considering addiction to specific substances. Any combination of four or more of the behaviors listed below justifies a psychiatric diagnosis of the individual as addicted.

DSM IV CRITERIA FOR ADDICTION

1. Preoccupation with the Chemical Between Periods of Use

Whether one is addicted to gambling, heroin, refined sugar, or cocaine, the experience is a roller-coaster ride of short-term satisfactions within a larger context of expectation, and frustration until the expectation is fulfilled. But when the addictive substance is illegal, the situation is more psychologically complex than otherwise. Involvement in illegal activities necessarily separates an individual in a fundamental way from people who are not similarly involved. From the point of view of an illegal addict, everyone with whom he comes in contact is either an insider or an outsider, either a person who can help him get drugs or one who can turn him over to the police. Everyone is either a friend or an enemy—and most people will be enemies, simply because of the nature of the activity. Addiction to an illegal substance therefore becomes the defining characteristic of the addict's life; it is the filter through which every encounter is viewed. This is not a function of the biochemistry of addiction or the intrinsic characteristics of the substances themselves. Not uncommonly, hospital patients become addicted to morphine or other painkillers during the course of their treatment, but they do not experience the isolating "me against the world" psychology of the illegal addict, for whom the antisocial and secretive aspects of addiction are a fundamental part of the experience. As one researcher puts it, "It is difficult for those who have never been addicted to [illegal] chemicals to understand the importance addicts attach to their drug of choice. . . . It is not uncommon for cocaine addicts to admit that, if forced to choose, they would choose cocaine over friends, lovers, or even family."

2. Using More of the Chemical Than Had Been Anticipated

"I can abstain but I cannot be temperate," declared the eighteenth-century scholar Samuel Johnson. Because he believed drunkenness was morally wrong, Johnson made tea rather than alcohol his chosen beverage—and he often drank sixty cups of tea in a day. But few "addictive personalities" have Johnson's level of insight into their own lack of control. No one begins taking drugs with the conscious intention of becoming an addict, and many people who "experiment" with illegal chemicals never become addicted. But it is characteristic of the addict to both overestimate his powers of self-control and underestimate the strength of his dependency. Until the fact of his addiction becomes undeniable, a drug user is quite likely to define an addict as "anyone who uses more drugs than I do."

3. Development of Tolerance to the Chemical

Dependence on narcotics and other controlled substances can develop rapidly, or even immediately in the case of strongly addictive drugs such as crack cocaine. Tolerance to the drug's effects can also quickly be achieved. During the last century, tincture of opium, known as laudanum, was commonly used as a pain reliever. The usual dose was twenty drops in a glass of water, repeated two or three times a day. The English poet Samuel Taylor Coleridge often used up to two full quarts of laudanum in a week, however, and Thomas De Quincey, author of *Confessions of an English Opium-Eater,* could consume up to eight thousand drops of the drug each day. This volume would have been quickly fatal to an inexperienced user.

The phenomenon of an addict's tolerance to drugs, with its obvious consequence of need for greater amounts, dictates that the habit must become a larger and larger part of his life. Once again, it's important to emphasize the isolating effect this search for drugs will have on the addict's relationship with mainstream society, and to point out that this isolation may be an important underlying intention of his addiction.

4. Characteristic Withdrawal Syndrome from the Chemical

All habit-forming drugs, including caffeine, sugar, and chocolate, produce withdrawal symptoms when their use is discontinued. Sometimes there is a violent shock to the system: for a heavy drinker, for instance, sudden withdrawal from alcohol can cause convulsions or even death. Novels and films have often depicted "cold turkey" withdrawal from heroin as intensely painful, and this is often the case. There is evidence, however, that the suffering that accompanies heroin withdrawal may be influenced by both the setting in which withdrawal takes place and by the expectations of the drug user. In therapeutic communities that discourage expression of suffering during withdrawal, recovering addicts experience much less discomfort than is common in other detoxification settings. In many cases, heroin withdrawal resembles a severe case of respiratory flu.

5. Use of the Chemical to Avoid or Control Withdrawal Symptoms

Despite the fact that withdrawal symptoms may be influenced by external factors, an addict's fear of an extremely difficult experience is often used to justify maintaining an addiction. Long after the pleasures of using a drug have become unattainable, the fear of painful withdrawal symptoms can motivate continued use.

6. Repeated Efforts to Stop or Cut Back Use of the Chemical

Despite the powers of self-control that addicts often ascribe to themselves, particularly in the first stages of their involvement with drugs, they often find themselves pulled in opposite directions during the course of addiction. On one side they are confronted by legal and moral condemnation from society in general. This demonization of the addict can of course be painful, but it may also arouse strong feelings of resistance and rebellion. On the other side, an addict usually joins a peer group of other drug users who encourage continued addiction, and whose friendship will be lost if drug use stops. During the course of even a single day an addict is exposed to literally hundreds of messages pointing him both toward and away from drugs. It should be no surprise, then, that addiction typically includes many failed attempts to stay away from drugs.

7. Intoxication at Inappropriate Times (Such as at Work), or When Withdrawal Interferes with Daily Functioning

Stress is difficult to define but easy to recognize. It's not really a well-defined sentiment like love or fear, but it's present in our lives at almost every moment, and it makes itself felt both physically and emotionally. I believe this pervasive stress is a unique phenomenon of modern life, and that nothing quite like it existed until relatively recently in human history. The prehistoric hunter trying to throw his spear at a saber-toothed tiger surely experienced acute fright; the medieval townsman threatened by the Plague undoubtedly was terrified; and the nineteenth-century farmers of the American plains must have felt helpless when their crops were threatened by drought—but these were at least feelings with clear causes and consciously perceived effects. In addition, religion in one form or another always provided an explanation for what was taking place, as well as solace to help cope with it. Today there's surely less terror than in the past, but there's more tension, a low to moderate level of background anxiety. For the addict, drugs can provide a chemical antidote to the problem of stress, an alternative reality whose very difficulties and dangers may be preferable to demands of everyday life. This doesn't mean that every heroin or cocaine user retreats for days at a time to a shooting gallery in some downtrodden area of the city; on the contrary, an addict may simply close the door to his office for a few moments. Once this method of tension reduction comes to be relied upon, however, it can take on a life of its own:

what began as a voluntary action to achieve a reassuring high becomes a compulsion to avoid a debilitating withdrawal.

8. Reduction in Social, Occupational, or Recreational Activities in Favor of Further Chemical Use

"It's so wonderful that you shouldn't even try it once." This quote, often cited in books on drug abuse, is ascribed to an anonymous heroin user trying to describe his initial experience with the drug. His paradoxical remark aptly expresses the power of certain drugs first to occupy and then completely pre-occupy a user's consciousness. The price of chemically induced ecstasy is increasing apathy to everything else. This has been demonstrated experimentally with laboratory rats who have become addicted to cocaine. In favor of obtaining the drug, the addicted animals will ignore any and all other stimuli, including food, water, and copulation with another rat. This narrowing of interest is a defining characteristic of drug addiction, and one of its most dangerous aspects.

9. Chemical Use Continues Despite Social, Emotional, or Physical Problems Related to Such Use

The writer William S. Burroughs, now more than eighty years old, has been a heroin addict for his entire adult life. In his novel entitled *Junky,* Burroughs wrote, "Junk is not a kick. It is a way of life." Both Burroughs's longevity and his output of creative work are certainly uncharacteristic of habitual drug users, but he is correct in describing drug use as more than simply a sensation produced by a series of chemical reactions in the body. Addiction is an all-encompassing orientation toward the world, and before it, everything else shrinks to unimportance. Perhaps this is even a latent intention in the mind of the drug user, for whom the physical self becomes all he knows, all he needs to know, and all he wants to know. The psychoanalytic interpretation of addiction traces its origins to unfulfilled dependency needs in the first stages of life, and in a sense the addict does regress to the stage of an infant sucking at a breast or a bottle. Nothing else matters, nothing else even exists, and the prospect that the source of nourishment might be removed is terrifying beyond expression.

DRUG USE AND THE DOSHAS

Vata

Addictive drug use begins as a kind of bargain in which immediate, short-term satisfaction is gained at the risk of serious long-term physical, emotional, and legal problems. Impatience—for sensation, for excitement, for peer acceptance—is a fundamental element of drug use in its early stages. And as addictive behavior continues, this impatience often assumes a frantic character, though it may later degrade into the numbness of apathy of advanced addiction. From an Ayurvedic viewpoint, the impatience that characterizes drug use is indicative of a Vata imbalance. Remember that Vata derives from the element of air, and like the wind this dosha is always changing direction and intensity, as if unable to rest or be satisfied. Ayurveda uses the Sanskrit word *sattva*, meaning purity, to describe the calm and clear-sighted awareness of the mind in its natural state. Drugs introduce an artificial, external influence on mental functioning. Depending on the drug, this influence may dull the senses or temporarily heighten them. But the ultimate effect is always to destabilize the mind's equilibrium and initiate the restlessness and unpredictability that characterizes Vata imbalance. Vata is also a very dry dosha, and the diuretic effect of many drugs can dry out the system, worsening the constipation and kidney problems that are typical of severely unbalanced Vata.

Use of amphetamines and other stimulants aggravate Vata severely and immediately. But even sedatives and opiates, despite their short-term effects, can have the same result. In any case, the various symptoms that accompany withdrawal from addictive drugs are basically Vata disorders, and they should be treated with Vata-pacifying techniques (presented in Part Three of this book).

Pitta

Pitta dosha derives from the element of fire, and in the Ayurvedic literature this dosha is frequently referred to through metaphors of heat. Pitta is responsible for the body's ability to digest and metabolize food, and most disorders of the digestive tract occur when Pitta's digestive fires are burning too hot or too low. It is significant that a word like *burnout* is often applied to the effects of long-term drug use, particularly of amphetamines and other stimulants, or of hallucinogens such as LSD or marijuana.

People with predominately Pitta constitutions are generally goal-oriented and demanding of themselves. When Pitta becomes unbalanced, they can become truly driven, and it's not uncommon for Pitta types to become involved with drugs in the belief that this will help them achieve their objectives. The French writer and philosopher Jean-Paul Sartre, for example, used amphetamines for many years in an effort to write as much as possible. Damage to the eyes is a common result of long-term involvement with amphetamines, and eventually Sartre lost his eyesight as a result of his drug use.

Kapha

Depression, lethargy, and a sedentary lifestyle are common indicators of Kapha imbalance. In an attempt to deal with these symptoms, Kapha types are often drawn to powerful stimulants for quick bursts of energy, or to opiates such as heroin or barbiturates such as Valium that simply exacerbate their inherent tendencies. In either case, natural sources of vitality are depleted rather than developed.

When a Kapha individual has been using drugs for some time, however, there is almost always a Vata imbalance, which must be addressed before the needs of the dominant dosha can be fulfilled. This may be difficult to recognize when excessive sleeping, eating, or other obvious symptoms of depression are present. Yet depression and anxiety are really two sides of the same coin, and an unbalanced Kapha type may sleep twelve hours a night without being truly relaxed even for a moment. For Kaphas as well as the other mind body types, the Vata balancing techniques described in Part Three should be the first step in restoring balance to the system after drug use.

7

TOBACCO ADDICTION

The role of tobacco in American life is one of the most hotly debated topics now before us. Unlike the consensus that exists regarding the hazards of addiction to an illegal drug such as heroin, or a legal but potentially dangerous drug such as alcohol, there is no general agreement on the status of tobacco in our society. Virtually all physicians condemn smoking, but there are powerful financial and political interests that defend and ardently promote tobacco use. And even though a warning from the Surgeon General appears on every pack of cigarettes, state and federal governments derive enormous revenues from cigarette taxes, which must necessarily introduce a certain level of ambivalence into any government attack on smoking. After all, tobacco remains a legal product, as tobacco companies are always eager to point out, and at the federal level there has never been any serious effort to change that status in many years. Yet smoking is directly implicated in the deaths of more than one thousand Americans every day.

Tobacco and our attitude toward it creates a dilemma that extends beyond the usual boundaries of a discussion of drug use. It encompasses fundamental issues of finance, demographics, and personal freedom in a way that other drugs do not. The production of the cocaine-producing coca plant or the opium-producing poppy are important to the economies of nations such as Peru and Afghanistan, and the United States government exerts pressure on those countries to end cultivation of those crops. Yet virtually all of our tobacco is legally grown within the borders of the United States despite the fact that smoking-related deaths number more than 400,000 each year, many more than those that result from all other forms of drug use. Even where the law does try to assert itself with regard to smoking, it has been largely ineffective—if not altogether ignored. Smoking by teenagers is illegal, for example, but more than three million teenagers are habitual smokers.

In this country virtually everyone who smokes knows that tobacco is dangerous to their health. When the "danger to your health" label on cigarette packages became a legal requirement, tobacco companies were happy to comply, believing that the presence of a "fair warning" would protect them from lawsuits by dying smokers. Whether it will in fact continue to protect them remains to be seen, but there is evidence that the warnings and other negative publicity regarding smoking are having an effect. Millions of Americans now quit smoking every year. It is also true, however, that many people find it impossible to stop smoking, and most of those who do quit (or never start) come from better educated and more affluent segments of society. Smoking is actually becoming more popular among certain demographic groups, such as young black males and teenage girls. There also seems to be a bright future for tobacco in other parts of the world. China, for example, with its more than one billion people, has a greater number of smokers than the entire population of the United States.

THE HISTORY AND APPEAL OF TOBACCO

As with alcohol, smoking has had a ceremonial function throughout its history. Smoking the "peace pipe" was a well-known ritual among some Native American tribes, and it was probably in this context that European explorers such as Sir Walter Raleigh first encountered tobacco. Raleigh is usually credited with the introduction of tobacco into England in the seventeenth century, though this may be historically inaccurate. Smoking had been known in Europe since Columbus's first expeditions to the New World, which took place a century before Raleigh's. In fact, a shipmate of Columbus was imprisoned "for the good of his soul" when he lit up a cigar upon returning to Spain. By the time he was released, smoking had become a popular pastime all over Europe.

It's interesting to note that from the beginning, smoking has provoked ambivalent and even contradictory responses from governments and even religious institutions. Smoking became punishable by death shortly after its first appearance in Germany. In Russia smokers could be sentenced to castration, and in America ten different states had laws against cigarettes as recently as 1909. But the popularity of smoking among the general population has always been strong. No harsh governmental measures have been able to slow the spread of the tobacco habit, and the impossibility of complete official suppression has become obvious. In contrast to today, the medical profession was initially less opposed to smoking than were the guardians of public morality; European physicians viewed tobacco as a powerful medicine rather than as a vice. But regardless of approval or disapproval from any official establishment, smoking has always become unstoppable wherever tobacco was introduced.

When cigarette-rolling machines were invented in the nineteenth century, a turning point in the history of tobacco was reached. Previously tobacco had been chewed, inhaled in the form of snuff, or smoked in pipes or as cigars, and the cumbersome nature of these methods had limited the volume of consumption. But even the earliest rolling machines could produce more than 100,000 cigarettes per day. Moreover, prerolled cigarettes were cheaper and easier to transport. They were also less long-lasting than other forms of tobacco, so a smoker was likely to light up more often. It's worth noting that the history of tobacco delivery systems have been paralleled by those of cocaine. Among large segments of the population, the use of powdered cocaine has been largely supplanted by crack, which has a low unit cost and a short duration of effect and is "convenient" to use.

Even this brief survey reveals an important aspect of smoking's appeal. From the first, it has been an easy form of transgression against official morality, a kind of risky business that was first practiced by "wild Indians." By the 1920s smoking was considered a mark of sophistication in the United States, in the same way that visiting a speakeasy allowed people to thumb their noses at authority during the same period. No doubt this is still a large part of tobacco's appeal to certain groups, especially adolescents. But smoking has also been a way of expressing comradeship, maturity, and a sense of personal style, as anyone who has ever watched a Humphrey Bogart or Bette Davis film will surely realize. Only in the past few decades has there been a real change in consciousness about tobacco among large segments of the population. Even these recent changes have been mostly confined to certain groups in the United States.

TOBACCO ADDICTION

Regardless of how tobacco was viewed in the past by the medical profession, today virtually all physicians warn their patients against smoking in the strongest possible terms. And although the tobacco industry continues to deny it, the addictive nature of smoking now seems beyond dispute.

Tobacco smoke contains about four thousand different chemical compounds—including carbon monoxide, ammonia, hydrogen cyanide, and formaldehyde—but it is common knowledge that smoking's principal psychoactive effects derive from nicotine. Researchers differ on the potency of nicotine's effects in comparison to substances such as cocaine or the amphetamines, but there is no doubt that nicotine is extremely addictive. Between 3 percent and 20 percent of people who ever try cocaine eventually become addicted, but between one-third to one-half of all "experimental" smokers become tobacco addicts. Research shows that an adolescent who smokes as few as four cigarettes has a 94 percent probability of continuing to use tobacco for a substantial part of his or her life.

There are many approaches to the treatment of tobacco and nicotine addiction. Virtually all of them are successful for certain smokers, while other people remain unable to quit no matter how many times they try. This suggests that the secret lies less in the treatment than in the mind and heart of the smoker—and I draw this conclusion from personal experience.

I began smoking when I was seventeen years old. Over the years I made many attempts to stop, but none were successful for long. I came to despise my smoking habit, and I was angry at myself for indulging in it. Very often I would furiously throw away the last five cigarettes in a pack while promising myself to quit. But within an hour or so I was always furtively opening a new pack. I saw that in some way the cycle of self-reproach and guilt was a mechanism that kept my habit alive, but this insight had no practical effect on my smoking. I simply acted out the sequence again and again. In Ayurvedic terms, my intention to quit was overwhelmed by the memories of smoking and the desires they ignited.

Then one evening I went to the ballet. As I sat there in the darkness admiring the graceful dancers, I could hear my own breathing coming in wheezes and gasps. The contrast made a powerful impression on me. Before me were superb athletes flying across the stage, and here I was struggling just to breathe.

The next day, as I was about to open a new pack of cigarettes, I felt more than the usual degree of guilt about my smoking. But I had learned by this time that guilt was not enough to break my addiction; in some mysterious way, guilt facilitated it. So instead of combining the toxic experience of smoking with my own toxic self-reproach, I let my thoughts return to the beautiful dancers I had seen the night before. By doing so, I finally discovered the way to break the chain of my addictive behavior, and I threw away my package of cigarettes. Over the new few weeks, I called upon the memory of the dancers whenever I felt the desire to smoke. I gave up trying to fight my addiction, and instead replaced it with a positive alternative.

I am not suggesting that this was a miraculous discovery on my part. Cognitive techniques and positive visualizations are the basis of numerous addiction therapies. But I had arrived at a point of sincere intention to quit smoking. By combining that intention with a vision of beauty and health, I was able to create a new sequence of memory, action, and desire. Remembering the dancers motivated me to the action of throwing away my cigarettes, and actually doing so was a positive experience that made me feel good about myself. The feeling was more powerful than whatever pleasure I got from smoking, and the desire to experience that feeling was stronger than my desire to smoke. I haven't had a cigarette in many years.

In telling how I managed to quit smoking, let me emphasize the importance of sincere intention. The ballet dancers were a very beautiful and inspiring sight, but no doubt I had seen other such sights during my years as a smoker. Suddenly, however, I was ready to become fully aware of those dancers. I was ready to see something wonderful that life has to offer, and to feel with my own wheezing breath how I had been denying it to myself.

Have you arrived at this point of sincere intention to stop smoking? If you have, I'm confident that the information in the next few pages can help you to do so.

QUITTING SMOKING: AN AYURVEDIC APPROACH

It's obvious from the worldwide popularity of smoking that this addiction is not limited to any well-defined group of people. From an Ayurvedic perspective, one can see how each of the three mind body types may be attracted to smoking for different reasons.

Vata types are likely to use tobacco as a way of dealing with restless energy. Handling a cigarette provides an outlet for the nervousness and inability to stay still that is characteristic of Vata when it is out of balance. Vatas may be more inclined to quit smoking than Pitta or Kapha types, but this is largely because Vatas are more inclined toward change in general. Although they may find it easier to quit, they are also more likely to start again. It's rare to meet a middle-aged Vata smoker who hasn't sworn off cigarettes at least three or four times.

For Pitta types, smoking expresses the urge toward power and self-assertion that is characteristic of this dosha. Pittas don't like to be bossed around; therefore, no amount of negative publicity about smoking is likely to have an effect. In fact, the whole experience of "playing with fire"—both literally and figuratively—has a strong appeal to the Pitta character. Pittas are also attached to highly scheduled and ritualized behaviors, and they're likely to feel the need for a cigarette very strongly at certain times of the day, especially after a meal.

Kapha-dominant individuals most often use smoking as an extension of their naturally slower-paced and contemplative lifestyle. Cigars hold a particular appeal for many Kapha men; the experience of settling into a comfortable chair with a big cigar is much more attractive to a Kapha sensibility than to a Vata's or Pitta's. Like Pitta types, Kaphas may stubbornly resist advice to quit smoking.

Regardless of their mind body type, I believe that anyone who wishes to stop smoking can benefit from the four-point technique described below. As it does in the case of alcohol, however, success depends on the spiritually grounded belief that you really want to replace smoking in your life with a different kind of pleasure, a higher order of satisfaction. Before you try to stop, examine what smoking has given to you, as well as what it has cost. Arrive at a point of sincere intention, and then use the method below as a practical guide for translating that intention into action.

Four Steps to Break the Smoking Habit

1. If you're like most smokers, you probably light your cigarettes, use them, and discard them without real awareness of what you're doing. Over the years, these behaviors have become deeply ingrained reflexes that occur almost automatically. So the first step toward quitting smoking is to become mindful of the fact that you *are* smoking. Before you light a cigarette, make a conscious effort to slow down the process. Look at the cigarette in your hand, and as you do so, listen to the internal signals of your body. Is this cigarette something that your body really wants? Or is the cigarette only a way of covering up something else that you're thinking or feeling? Even if you decide that you really do want to smoke the cigarette, listening to your body will slow down the process and shut off your "automatic pilot." Though it may seem strange, when you're first learning this technique it can be useful to watch yourself in a mirror as you prepare to smoke. This will help you be-

come a conscious observer of yourself during the critical moments when you're about to light up. Always remember that an important step in dealing with any addiction is to eliminate urgent behavior and replace it with full awareness. Just by becoming mindful of what you're doing, you can often make rapid progress in breaking the habit of smoking.

2. As with drinking and other addictive behaviors, the impulse to smoke is often triggered by a wide range of cues and signals. Many people unconsciously light a cigarette when talking on the telephone or while drinking a cup of coffee. Try to make smoking an isolated, independent activity. This will facilitate the mindfulness discussed in step 1. Even if you continue to smoke for a period of time, you will at least be aware of what you're doing. You will also become aware of the unpleasant sensations associated with the activity.

3. Once you have developed a degree of mindfulness about your habit, begin to introduce some new thoughts into the process of smoking a cigarette. For me, this was the visualization of the ballet dancers, but you can use any deeply pleasant thought or memory. It must have definite spiritual significance for you, however, and you must access the memory with sincere intention. It's difficult to define precisely what this means, but you will intuitively know the difference between a thought that takes you into the realm of the spirit and one that is devoid of spiritual significance. Focus on this thought or memory. Allow it to overshadow your desire to smoke. What aspirations does it awaken in your mind? What feelings does it create in your body? Let yourself experience these things with mindful awareness until the desire for a cigarette has passed.

4. Focusing on a spiritually significant thought or memory is really a basic form of meditation—a first step in the profound adventure of consciousness. Meditation is

discussed more fully in Part Three of this book, along with other techniques for getting in touch with your higher self. These techniques are tremendously useful and perhaps even indispensable for ending addiction of any kind. In fact, I have never encountered a person who regularly meditated, practiced yoga, or followed a related spiritual discipline who was also engaged in addictive behaviors. *In my opinion, the only lasting solution to smoking or addiction of any kind lies in the discovery of your true spiritual nature.*

8

FOOD ADDICTION

During the years he spent at the Institute for Advanced Study in Princeton, New Jersey, Albert Einstein was known to become deeply absorbed in his scientific contemplations. In his history of the institute, *Who Got Einstein's Office?*, Edward Regis recounts an incident that took place one afternoon when the great physicist was walking alone near his house. When he encountered a younger colleague from the institute, the two men talked for a few minutes and then were about to go their separate ways. But Einstein hesitated.

"Excuse me, but I have one final question," he said. "When we stopped to talk a moment ago, was I walking toward my house, or away from it?"

Many people would have been surprised by an inquiry like this, but people who worked with Einstein had learned to expect anything. "You were walking away from your house," the younger professor replied. "I'm certain of it."

"Excellent," Einstein said with a smile. "That means I've already eaten my lunch." And he continued on toward his office.

Perhaps Einstein really didn't care about food, at least as long as he got enough of it. But if he was not able to eat for a few days, you can be certain that Einstein's thoughts would turn away from the mysteries of time and space and toward the best way to get a peanut butter sandwich. No one is really indifferent to eating—we're all "addicted" to it. But nature intends that this should be a positive addiction in every way, and Ayurveda places great emphasis on the sensations and pleasures associated with taking nutritious food into our bodies, as well as its importance to our health.

It is unfortunate that our society, which has eliminated the problem of hunger more successfully than any other culture in history, is also home to a vast array of eating disorders. All of these disorders are dangerous, and in extreme forms they are life threatening. There is also evidence that the situation is becoming worse, especially with regard to the overweight problem throughout the population.

Statistically, there's an excellent chance that you have personal familiarity with excessive weight gain. It is estimated that half the total adult population of the United States goes on a diet at some point during any given year. The weight-loss industry is annually a $30 billion business. Yet the weight of the average American continues to rise, and seats in new baseball stadiums are now made half an inch wider than they used to be.

To some extent, this collective expansion has a technological explanation. People just don't do as much physical labor as they used to, so they don't burn as many calories. Also, the content of many people's diets is different from that of their parents, with more refined sugar and additional grams of fat. But despite these external variables, if you're seriously overweight there's a good chance that your eating habits include elements of addictive behavior.

This is an area in which Ayurvedic insights and techniques can be particularly effective. To the ancient seers who created

Ayurveda, the act of eating and the choice of what to eat were of the greatest significance. The principles they laid down, which have been refined through the centuries, are notable both for their good common sense and for their congruence with current research on eating disorders. Quite simply, they work. The information and techniques presented in this chapter can quickly help you put an end to compulsive or addictive eating habits. They can be the first steps toward finding true pleasure in eating and real joy in life.

EATING AND ADDICTIVE BEHAVIOR

Newborn babies cry. They don't know what they're crying about, they just know *something's wrong, something hurts*. But the mother of a newborn knows that the baby is hungry, and that's easy enough to fix. As the baby's lips close around the nipple and the milk begins to flow, the *something* that was wrong begins to feel right. Where there was pain, there is now pleasure. Again, the baby doesn't understand the mechanisms of this. He or she just knows that eating makes things feel better—and this is a connection that no human being is likely to forget.

Nature ordained that discomfort caused by hunger would be diminished by food. But what about discomfort caused by pressures at work? Or by loneliness or anger? What about the emotional pain caused by being seriously overweight—can *that* be alleviated by eating? Of course, the short-term answer is yes, just as these problems can also be momentarily banished by an alcoholic drink or a heroin injection. But these palliatives are really regressions to a state of infantile dependency, attempts to recapture the sensation that a crying baby experiences when he or she just suddenly and miraculously feels better. Unfortunately, this is one area in which we really "can't go home again." With regard to food addiction, the lesson to be drawn is this: when you're an adult, don't try to deal with your problems the way you did when you were an infant.

If you're unhappy with your work, you should have a talk with your supervisor. If you're not satisfied with a relationship, you should express your feelings. And if you're really hungry, regardless of whether you're overweight, by all means eat. But if you're not hungry, don't eat.

If you're not hungry, don't eat! I want to emphasize that point because it really is the key to overcoming food addiction. In our discussions of alcohol, drugs, and tobacco, I've tried to give attention to the pleasures of those substances as well as the dangers they present. But is there really a need to highlight the pleasures of eating? Certainly there are people, like Albert Einstein, who have a lot of other things on their minds, but for most of us eating is a great source of happiness. But when eating becomes your *principal* source of happiness, or even your only source of happiness, problems are bound to arise. As it is in the case of other addictive behaviors, the challenge in overcoming food addiction lies in finding positive, truly pleasurable alternatives. It isn't just a matter of eating less, but also of doing something joyful instead. In Part Three of this book, you'll find some suggestions regarding diet, as well as some ideas to help you discover new sources of joy in your life. You'll have plenty of chances to explore these new sources, because all the time you've spent eating when you're not hungry will now become available. Remember: *If you're not hungry, don't eat!*

This won't necessarily be easy, at least not at first, and it will require some focused attention. But by learning to listen to your body and to understand its messages, you can turn this single sentence into a life-changing principle.

If you've been struggling with food addiction for some time, you may literally have forgotten how to identify genuine hunger for food from some other craving "in disguise." Real hunger is a signal from inside your body that your system is now prepared to ingest and metabolize food. Many other needs, dissatisfactions, or yearnings may cause you to put food in your mouth, but your digestive system will not be able to effectively process that food and it will be stored as fat. In learning to distinguish real hunger, you must be mindful. As with cigarette smoking, you must learn to transform previously automatic, reflexive eating behaviors into conscious, mindful ones—and there is a surprisingly simple technique that can help you do this. Follow it for the next two weeks and not only will you be eating more wisely, you'll also be listening to your body in a way that is fundamental to Ayurveda's approach to human health.

Before you begin to eat, whether it's a mid-morning snack or a formal dinner, place your hand on your stomach and mindfully assess your hunger level. Is your stomach telling you that you're really hungry, or is the desire for food coming from somewhere else? What are you actually feeling? What is it that you *really* want?

Once you do start eating, from time to time place your hand on your stomach again to ascertain your level of satisfaction. Eat to a point of comfortable satiety, but don't feel that you have to go on eating until you can't possibly swallow another bite. The stomach is not like the gas tank of a car that needs to be filled up whenever you stop at a station. Ayurveda teaches that the human digestive system is like a fire: too much fuel can smother it. It's best to eat to no more than three-quarters of your capacity, and with practice you can learn to accurately identify this point. Try placing your hand over your stomach several times a day to estimate your hunger level. You may even want to keep a written record, noting how you feel at various times and how your eating behavior reflects this.

Awareness, intention, mindfulness, and learning to focus on the inner intelligence of your body as well as the supreme wisdom of the universe, which expresses itself in you, are the guiding principles of healthy eating. No one can tell you how much you "should" weigh or how much you "should" eat. You really know these things yourself. You just need to become aware of your body's inner wisdom.

ADDICTIVE EATING AND THE DOSHAS

Vata, Pitta, and Kapha express themselves through eating in characteristic ways. But as with other addictions, there is usually a Vata imbalance if addictive eating behavior has been taking place for any length of time. Keep this in mind as you look over the descriptions that follow. Even if your results on the mind body questionnaire indicate that you're a Kapha or a Pitta type, pay particular attention to the information on Vata eating habits. In Part Three, you'll find suggestions for a diet that's specially designed to pacify Vata.

Vata

Irregularity is a hallmark of Vata eating behavior, especially when the dosha is out of balance. Sometimes Vata types will resolve to follow a very well-organized diet; they may even become suddenly interested in nutritional benefits of various foods as well as possible dangers from pesticides and other additives. However, they may just as suddenly feel an extreme craving for something completely different—ice cream, cookies, red meat, chocolate bars—and unbalanced Vatas find these temptations difficult to resist. This feast-or-famine behavior is in some ways comparable to the alcoholic binge drinker, and it creates a sense that one's life is out of control. Paradoxically, Vata types can also be consistent or even constant eaters. Like chain-smoking, popping things in their mouths all day is simply a manifestation of general anxiety.

Pitta

As in every other area of life, Pitta eating is characterized by a need for organization and predictability. Most Pitta types like to eat three meals a day and prefer to have those meals at exactly the same time. The composition of the meals may be less important than their constancy. Philosopher Ludwig Wittgenstein, whose ideas reflect the Pitta outlook carried to its limit, once remarked, "I don't care what I eat as long as it's the same thing every day." Most Pittas would probably not go that far, but they do tend to get upset if their eating patterns—or any other patterns—of their lives become disrupted. When such disruptions occur, as they inevitably do, the anger that lies just below the surface of the Pitta personality is likely to burst forth. Many Pitta food addicts use eating as an expression of rage—they are literally "swallowing their anger." Without being consciously aware of it, out-of-balance Pitta types may actually see habitual overeating as an act of rebellion, an expression of defiance against the world's injustice.

Kapha

The innate sensuality of the Kapha nature can easily express itself through eating, and when other sources of pleasure are denied or ignored, out-of-balance Kapha types can easily become food addicts. Combining aspects of the Vata binge eater with a Pitta's demand for three square meals a day, Kaphas can eat almost constantly, both at mealtimes and whenever they happen to see something tempting in a bakery or delicatessen. Inherent in the Kapha personality is a desire to avoid confrontation, both with other people and with emotional issues within themselves. Food can serve to "cover up" or "smother" these intense emotions, but as this does not really deal with the feelings at their core, a sense of depression can result. In a vicious circle, out-of-balance Kaphas may try to deal with their depression by eating even more. It's important to note that food addiction often gives rise to serious health problems in people of this dosha. Diabetes and obesity, both exacerbated by the Kapha's love for sweets, are two very common conditions.

A HEALTHY DIET: AN ALTERNATIVE TO FOOD ADDICTION

In the West, foods are categorized according to their fat content and the number of calories they contain. In recent years we've also made a distinction between so-called organic foods and those that are highly processed and contain various additives. But although we use these words when we decide what to eat, it's unlikely that many people really know what the terms mean. Most people simply rely on the notion that "less is more"; in other words, fewer calories and lower fat content means good. Depending on the needs of the individual, this assumption may not always be true. If you need immediate and sustained energy, for example, high-calorie foods can be very beneficial.

Ayurveda relies on a highly experiential system for classifying foods. It involves no numbers, grams, or calories per ounce. Instead, Ayurvedic categories are based on how the foods actually taste when we put them into our mouths. This taste-based system is highly developed, and Ayurveda recognizes six distinct categories. By becoming familiar with the six tastes and by following the important Ayurvedic principle of including all six tastes in every meal, you can eliminate many of the cues that underlie addictive eating behavior. You'll enjoy your food more as well.

The six tastes are: *sweet, sour, salty, pungent, bitter,* and *astringent.* No doubt four of them are quite familiar, but pungent and astringent may seem new. Here are some common examples of all six tastes:

- Sweet: sugar, honey, rice, wheat, bread, milk, cream
- Sour: cheese, yogurt, lemons, plums, and other sour fruits
- Salty: any food to which salt has been added
- Pungent: all spicy, hot-tasting food, including chili peppers, salsa, cayenne, and ginger
- Bitter: spinach, romaine lettuce, and all leafy greens
- Astringent: beans, lentils, pomegranates, apples, pears, and cabbage

The sweet taste is by far the most popular in most Western countries, and it deserves special attention. Our "sugar addiction" often begins in early childhood, with commercial breakfast foods and candy bars, and for many people the craving for sweets lasts throughout their lives. Moreover, certain foods that are not sweet themselves nevertheless create a desire for sweets: eating red meat, for instance, often makes many people wish for a sugary dessert. As you implement an Ayurvedic approach to your diet, begin by evaluating the role sweets play in your eating habits. There's a good chance this one taste accounts for a large portion of your total food intake. To reduce a craving for sweets, try taking a little honey as a substitute for foods containing refined sugar. Because sugar creates desire for more sugar, taking honey at breakfast can help break a chain of sugary foods that might otherwise last all day.

Once you become aware of the sweet foods in your diet, you can begin to notice the presence or absence of the other tastes as well. With a little effort, you can plan your meals to include all or most of them, and you may be surprised by the dramatic effect this can have not only on your eating habits but on your life as a whole. Tastes can directly influence our emotions, which is evident even in the language we use to describe them; phrases such as "sweet memories," "bitter grief," and "sour grapes" are a few examples. They can also influence our physical state. Some hot spices can literally cause us to break out in a sweat, while cooler tastes such as mint can bring an overall sense of refreshment.

By including all the tastes in your meals, you can make them a more complete and satisfying experience both emotionally and nutritionally. A good Ayurvedic cookbook can help you plan your meals, and even the planning will make you more mindful of what you eat. I especially recommend the cookbook *A Simple Ceremony*, by Ginna Bragg and my colleague David Simon, M.D.

THE LIMITS OF BEHAVIORISM

Because eating disorders are so prevalent in our society, they've been the subject of intense scrutiny from both the scientific and the business communities. Immense profits await anyone who can offer a quick and easy way to control overeating, and there have been instances in which great successes have taken place in this area, at least in the short run. Once again, however, I want to emphasize the importance of *sincere intention* and *spiritual awareness* in any permanent solution to any addictive behavior.

I think the following story well illustrates the limits of a purely mechanistic approach to a food addiction. It is told by Andrew Weil, M.D., and Winifred Rosen in their excellent book, *From Chocolate to Morphine*.

A young woman had been deeply addicted to chocolate for a number of years. She absolutely had to have chocolate several times a day, and her life had literally become organized around this compulsion. If she awakened in the middle of the night and found herself without any chocolate in her home, she did not hesitate to get into her car and find an all-night supermarket in order to satisfy her need. After several years of this, she went to a clinic that specialized in treating eating disorders. The treatment proved to be not at all what she might have expected, but it was quite effective nonetheless. After making a commitment to attend ten sessions at the clinic, she was asked to sit in front of a large mirror. She was then given a supply of chocolate candy and a device was attached to her wrist that continuously transmitted a low-intensity, completely painless electric shock. For thirty minutes, she was to watch herself in the mirror as she ate the chocolate candy—but instead of swallowing the candy, she was instructed to spit each mouthful onto a paper plate. At first this procedure seemed somewhat absurd, and through the first seven sessions it had no effect. The young woman's addiction to chocolate remained strong as ever, and it was only because she had paid for ten sessions that she continued going to the clinic. After the eighth session, however, she began to notice diminished interest in chocolate, and, though it seemed incredible, her compulsion completely vanished by the end of the tenth session. Several years have passed and her chocolate addiction has not returned. Unfortunately, she then became addicted to cake!

My purpose in retelling this story is to show both the possibilities and the limits of a purely behaviorist approach to food addiction, and in fact to any addiction. Such approaches may certainly be ingenious. They may even be effective in dealing with the problem in a narrowly defined sense. But the addictive behavior is only being suppressed, and the spiritual needs that underlie it remain unsatisfied. The basis of the addiction remains untouched, and almost inevitably it finds yet another avenue to express itself.

The real source of any addiction, and the real opportunity for positive development in any human being, is accessible only through the Spirit. In this connection, I often cite the example of someone who hears Beethoven's music played on a radio and then begins dismantling the radio in an effort to find Beethoven. But Beethoven isn't in the radio, and the brain, the central nervous system, the digestive system, and all the "nuts and bolts" of the body are not really "nuts and bolts" at all. They are expressions of the higher self. They are reachable through sincere intention. And no matter how entrenched an addiction may seem, it can be made to vanish before the spiritual power within you.

9

OTHER SOURCES OF

ADDICTION

So far we've dealt with substance-related addictions, and we've seen how they've been part of human history almost from the beginning. Contemporary society, however, is an environment in which whole new categories of addictive behavior have come into being. In this chapter we'll look briefly at three examples of these uniquely "modern" addictions. Although they are not based on substance abuse and are not directly life threatening, these behavior patterns have all the characteristics of classic addiction. They may, however, be even more difficult to recognize and confront. Addiction to work, to destructive relationships, and to television don't involve any illegal activity. They are addictive in the sense that they can occupy a disproportionately large area of a person's life—or perhaps even all of it.

WORK ADDICTION

Everyone knows the word *workaholic,* but I don't think it's really an accurate term. Workaholic implies an analogy between addiction to work and addiction to alcohol. Yet the two addictions are really quite different.

For example, we could describe a person who drinks too much as being "out of control." An alcoholic can't control his or her behavior with respect to drinking. As the addiction to alcohol progresses, this lack of control eventually expresses itself in obvious ways: trembling, falling down, car accidents, difficulty in sleeping or waking up, and all sorts of other signs that the person's physical, intellectual, and emotional guidance systems aren't operating properly. This may even be a kind of unconscious goal or strategy on the part of some alcoholics, one which is related to the psychoanalytic view of alcoholism as an attempt to deal with unsatisfied needs that go back to infancy. When he loses control, the alcoholic returns to a condition in which other people are called upon to take care of him. Others may or may not agree to do this, but the out-of-control alcoholic is asking for, or even demanding, assistance in basic life tasks.

The so-called workaholic is doing something very different. While alcoholism can often be an almost childlike way of reaching out to people, working all the time is a turning away from others. It is withdrawal into an area of life in which control is called for, and in which mastery is held in high regard. Beneath the behavior of an alcoholic there may be an underlying infantile fantasy, but the workaholic portrays himself or herself as a *total adult.*

The control fantasy that gives rise to work addiction almost always derives from a sense that other areas of life are beyond one's control. More specifically, workaholics often feel unequipped to deal with the stresses of family relationships: "Don't bother me, I've got to work" seems like a respectable or even an admirable way out. "Mow the lawn," "Pay the bills," "Wash the dog," and "Don't forget our anniversary" are all silenced by, *"I'm working! This is really important!"*

Some years ago I was involved in the case of a young girl who required prolonged hospitalizations and several major surgeries. Her treatment ultimately proved successful, but she spent many weeks at a time in a pediatric ward where the only entertainment was a walk down the hall or a visit to the ward's playroom. Although the family's home was in a small city some distance from the hospital, the girl's mother was with her every day and her father flew in to visit every weekend.

There was another girl in an adjacent room whose father virtually never made an appearance; it was, apparently, entirely the mother's responsibility to provide companionship for this child during her hospitalization. This drew the attention of everyone on the floor since the father was a well-known and powerful man in the entertainment industry, and his multimillion-dollar transactions were scrupulously reported by the press.

During my visits to the hospital, I found myself becoming angrier and angrier at the big deal-maker who couldn't find time to see his own daughter. It was hard to believe he was behaving this way, and I found myself imagining what I would say to him if I ever encountered him. Of course, I did eventually encounter him. He made one visit to his child and I happened to be present at the time. All the anger I had felt toward this man quickly evaporated when I actually saw him, because it was clear to me that he was in a state of terror. The signifiers of his power—the way he was dressed, his portable telephone, his wristwatch, his hairstyle—all meant nothing in the hospital environment. Here he was called upon to relinquish his own self-importance, and in some basic way this overwhelmed him. He evaporated. He felt invisible. When he departed, there was a noticeable lowering of tension in the air, which I'm sure was highly therapeutic for his daughter.

I've always felt that seriousness is a quite toxic state of mind, and the workaholic has a deep investment in seriousness: work is serious, he's serious about work, therefore he should be taken very seriously. But in fact all the work is a retreat from responsibilities that may be more truly serious than a workaholic wants to admit. If you're devoting every waking minute to your work, ask yourself whether this is really a necessity, or a choice. What might you be called upon to do if your work weren't so supremely important? Once you become comfortable in other areas of your life, you'll no longer need the refuge that work has provided.

SEX ADDICTION

Sex has been so stigmatized and vilified throughout Western history that we should probably be very careful in passing judgment on anyone's sexual behavior. Yet there's no doubt that some people become so preoccupied with sex that it causes difficulties in their lives. We can refer to this as sexual addiction, but we should be aware of the dangerous tendency to judge harshly any sexual behavior that differs from our own. On the other hand, there's no escaping the fact that sexual conduct is an important issue, as well as a target for moralists.

Sexuality is a fascinating and extremely complex subject. In the small space we're able to give to sexual addiction here, I'll refer to two states of being that seem to result in this behavior. In the first of these, there is an overstimulated emotional and physical condition from which release is desperately sought. In the second, there is an almost opposite kind of existence: a flattened landscape badly in need of some excitement.

The human nervous system cannot experience both pain and orgasm at the same time. Since pain, both physical and emotional, is absent at the moment of sexual climax, it follows that more climaxes mean less pain. I mention this because I've noticed that many sex addicts are in severe pain. Quite often it is physical pain, particularly in men, and I've observed that men with chronic health problems become preoccupied with sex disproportionately often. The great poet Lord Byron, for example, had a clubfoot and endured severe pain throughout his short life. By today's standards, Byron would definitely be considered a sex addict.

Sex can also provide an escape from emotional as well as physical pain, not only at the moment of orgasm but throughout all the stages of search and seduction. Quite often a sex addict really wants and needs to be *liked,* but since he or she feels excluded from this, the alternative is to be *loved,* at least in a physical sense. For people who become sexual addicts to escape pain, sex provides a kind of tranquillity. These people's systems are chronically overstimulated—in Ayurvedic terms, Vata is severely out of balance—and the purpose of sex is more to dampen their internal fires than to ignite them.

A second category of sexual addiction results from a kind of understimulation that culminates in depression. Some escape has to be found from an apparently purposeless existence, and sex seems to provide it. I once had an acquaintance who was able to end his sexual addiction when this suddenly became clear to him. He had one of those spiritual moments that I believe are almost a requirement for breaking free of addictive behaviors. This man had inherited enough money so that he could devote all his time to pursuing women. He preferred affairs that demanded lots of ingenuity, arduous pursuit, and transcontinental travel. One day he was on a boat searching the Greek islands for a certain woman when he was hit by a stunning realization. For the first time, he saw it wasn't the woman he really wanted—it was the intensity, the planning, the *purpose* that she gave to his life. In the absence of sex, and all that sex entailed, he really had not been able to find anything else for himself to do.

Sex can mean everything or it can mean nothing. Perhaps it's best if it means something somewhere in between.

TELEVISION ADDICTION

Television was invented in the 1920s, and within ten years the technology of the medium was fully developed. Fifty years ago, television could do virtually everything it is able to do today, but the Second World War delayed its distribution to the public. When TV finally did become widely available in the late 1940s and early 1950s, it almost instantly became hugely popular. Once television sets began appearing in homes, important changes began in the lifestyles of millions of people. Those transformations have continued, and accelerated, right up to the present.

Today millions of Americans watch television for as much as eight hours a day, but does television watching really meet the diagnostic criteria of addictive behavior? A great deal of evidence indicates that it does. We have seen, for example, that the presence of withdrawal symptoms is one of the defining characteristics of addiction, and television clearly causes such symptoms. There have been two studies in which families were paid several hundred dollars a month for *not* watching television, but both studies had to be terminated prematurely when the subjects simply could not endure the deprivation. Other research indicates that, as with heroin, television withdrawal symptoms for serious viewers are most severe after five to seven days. The symptoms include feelings of aggression, anxiety, depression, and difficulties in dealing with newly available free time. Subjects who succeeded in keeping their eyes off the screen for a week then began to feel comfortable in their new way of life.

Another marker of addictive behavior is the sense of guilt that accompanies it, and which somehow seems to fuel the addiction rather than suppress it. In a study of leisure-time activities, tele-vision was the only one that evoked feelings of guilt. Other leisure activities created more pleasure the longer they were pur-sued, but television produced guilt rather than enjoyment.

There are many other parallels between habitual television watching and other addictions. Like cigarette smoking, it is es-pecially prevalent among the poor. Like heroin and other nar-cotics, it offers a fantasy world that over time can become a kind of alternate reality for the viewer. And like all addictions, it derives from the absence of genuine pleasure, joy, and fulfill-ment in other areas of life.

Why do people watch television for many hours each day? Research among habitual TV watchers has yielded four basic motivations: a wish to escape the boredom of their daily lives; a desire to have something they can talk about with other peo-ple; the pleasure of seeing people and events on the screen with which they can compare their own experiences; and keeping in touch with the news and events of the world. With the possible exception of the final one, each of these reasons for watching television is clearly related to loneliness and de-privation in the real life of the addicted viewer. When there is real beauty and adventure in your life, there is no need to dra-matize it by comparing yourself with characters on sitcoms or soap operas. But when there is only boredom in your daily routine, the prefabricated adventures of stock characters pro-vide an alternative.

An eminent psychoanalyst has defined boredom as "desire for desire." We're bored when we know we want something, but we don't quite know what that something is. Rather than looking for an answer among the programs on television, we should learn to recognize our true needs and find ways to sat-isfy them in the things we do every day. This does not require large sums of money or great intelligence or extraordinary tal-ent. Everyone has the ability to create genuine pleasure in their lives: we all did it as children, and though we may become estranged from it for many years, the power to create joy always remains with us, waiting to be rediscovered and explored.

One of the interesting things about television is the way it makes things smaller. Almost anything that appears on the screen is almost always reduced in size from what it is in the real world. In a sense, this is true of all addictive behaviors: they diminish our experience of the world. Addictions demand time, money, intellectual energy, and even love that could and should find many other avenues of expression. In the remaining chapters of this book, we'll look at some Ayurvedic techniques for expanding your ability to participate fully in the world and for experiencing the joy of your own spirit.

PART THREE

RESTORING BALANCE

Earlier I suggested that an addict is a seeker of joy, but one who has been looking in the wrong places and has become sidetracked there, perhaps for many years. We explored some of those side roads in Part Two. But all this was in preparation for the ideas and techniques presented in the pages that follow. In other words, wherever you may have been in the past, now you've "come to the right place"!

Despite their apparent differences, the topics I will cover in Part Three—meditation, exercise, Vata balancing diet, and joyful daily activities—are really diverse approaches to the same goal. If I were to describe that goal in the fewest possible words, I would call it *perfect health*. The Ayurvedic concept of perfect health is founded on the idea that body, mind, and spirit are truly one—and therefore perfect health is achieved when the physical, intellectual, and spiritual sides of our nature are working together efficiently and harmoniously. The purpose of the material in Part Three, and the purpose of Ayurveda as a whole, is to help you discover, use, and enjoy the tools that nature gave you for making that goal a reality.

Your results on the mind body questionnaire indicate your dominant dosha. In a basic sense, this is who you are physically and emotionally. The balance point of your nature was set at your birth, and in Sanskrit this balance point is called your *prakriti,* a word that literally means "nature." But stresses of all kinds can cause deviations from the natural condition of harmony in your system, resulting in the state of imbalance that is called *vakriti.* Although your underlying nature has not changed and your dominant dosha remains the same, your currently unbalanced condition can mean that another dosha is presently exerting an unduly strong influence. When addictive behavior has been present for some time, the excessively influential dosha is virtually always Vata—and it's important to note that even individuals who are natural Vata types can also be subject to Vata imbalances. Because of Vata's destabilizing influence on most people who have a history of addiction, the techniques in this section of the book are designed to pacify Vata dosha. Once this has been accomplished and your system moves closer to its natural state of prakriti, you can make further adjustments in your diet, your exercise routine, and your other Ayurvedic practices so that they are no longer oriented specifically toward balancing Vata. To learn more about this, I suggest you consult my book *Perfect Health,* or arrange for a consultation with an Ayurvedic physician.

Although all the material in Part Three can be enormously beneficial in dealing with addictive behavior, I want to emphasize the special importance of meditation. All addictions have one thing in common: their power depends on something external, something out there in the world, something extrinsic to the individual self. It may be a powder or a liquid or a machine, but it's not something you were born with—you've got to find it and buy it and drink it or swallow it. In contrast, meditation comes entirely from within. You already have everything you need to meditate. You had it when you came into the world. No one can sell it to you, and no one can take it away from you. Meditating is the opposite, the antithesis, of addictive behavior, and I urge you to give particular attention to the chapter on meditation that follows.

10

MEDITATION

We have seen how an addiction can be an attempt to serve a variety of needs, and we have seen how those needs can be understood in terms of an individual's mind body type. A Vata-dominant person may drink in order to relax. For a Pitta type, drinking can provide an opportunity to test and demonstrate self-mastery, while for a Kapha, drinking can be a manifestation of depression and withdrawal from other people. From an Ayurvedic perspective, the purpose of meditating is quite different from any of these goals, despite the widespread belief that meditation is basically a way to relax. In fact, one of the most remarkable aspects of meditation is its power to encompass seemingly disparate states of mind in a single experience—an experience that I describe as *restful alertness*.

The word *restful* probably seems straightforward enough, but what about *alertness*? Alertness to what? To answer this, we must look for a moment at the way our minds operate during our everyday lives. Perhaps the most obvious thing about how our minds work is the way they're *always* working. One thought leads to another in a chain that stretches from morning to night. Memories, desires, aspirations toward pleasure, and aversions from pain—for most people there's never an internally quiet moment, and even the suggestion of a halt in the "stream of consciousness" might seem a bit frightening.

Although the ceaseless activity of thought is something we're all familiar with, there's another, very different experience that most people have also shared, and by understanding it we can begin to grasp the meaning of restful alertness.

Right now, try to remember what it's like to awaken from a deep sleep. As you open your eyes from such a sleep, it may take a moment to remember where you are. For a second or two, you may not even know *who* you are. But gradually the machinery of your thoughts and senses begins to take hold: your personality, your memories, your obligations for the coming day, your feelings for the many different people in your life—all these fall back into place. Still, there's no denying that, for a moment, there was a "you" that was somehow apart from you. There was a "you" that existed purely as an observer, and that was off the track of thoughts and feelings that carries you through the day. Meditation can help you first to acknowledge the existence of that magical silent observer and then to gain access to it on a regular basis. Gradually, you'll learn to use that state of restful alertness as a kind of internal compass or centering point, a place of strength from which the influence of Spirit can spread to all areas of your life. As this begins to happen, the mental static of your daily thoughts will sharpen into the clear harmony that is your true nature.

Over the years, many studies have demonstrated the benefits of meditation to people in all conditions and walks of life, from cancer patients to professional athletes. The simple but powerful technique presented here can be of great benefit in restoring balance to your system and in getting in touch with your higher self.

BREATHING MEDITATION

Despite what you may have expected, many forms of meditation require no special expertise or instruction. The method presented here requires nothing more than a focused but detached awareness of the process of respiration; in other words, an attitude of *mindfulness* toward your breathing.

If this seems almost too easy, consider what really takes place whenever you draw a breath. With each inhalation, your body takes in tens of billions of atoms, tiny fragments of the universe that over the centuries have passed through countless numbers of other living beings and will continue to do so long after you are no longer here. In this sense, breathing is literally an act of sharing. It is a biological process that puts us in touch with the past and the future of our own species, and with all other living beings as well.

To appreciate the significance of breathing at the level of your own daily experience, consider the close relationship between the way you breathe and how you feel, both physically and emotionally. When you're frightened or exhausted, the pace of your breathing speeds up while the quality of each breath becomes shallower. But when you're relaxed, you breathe deeply and regularly, and you feel even more relaxed as a result. Breathing is the link between the biological and spiritual elements of our nature. And breathing meditation is a powerful tool for uniting those elements into a single wholeness of being.

Practice breathing meditation twice each day, in the morning and in the early evening. Each session should last from twenty to thirty minutes. As you become more experienced with meditation, your mind will become quiet and you'll gain access to the state of restful alertness that precedes everyday thought. The stresses of addictive behavior will naturally diminish, because a new source of peace, joy, and inner strength has been revealed.

Breathing Meditation

1. Set aside a time when you can be free from interruptions and responsibilities.
2. In a quiet space free from traffic noise or other distractions, sit comfortably on the floor or in a straight-backed chair. Close your eyes.
3. Breathe normally, but begin to focus your attention on the rhythm of your breath. Without trying to control or influence it in any way, become aware of air entering and leaving your body.
4. If you notice your breath becoming faster or slower, or even stopping completely for a moment, just observe this with neither resistance nor encouragement. Let the normal rhythm return by itself.
5. If your thoughts distract you, or you feel yourself becoming unfocused in any way, don't resist. Just allow your attention to come back naturally to your breathing.
6. Continue this meditation for twenty to thirty minutes. Then, still sitting with your eyes closed, allow another few minutes for gradual return to everyday consciousness.
7. Slowly open your eyes and let your senses take in the sights and sounds around you.

PRIMORDIAL SOUND MEDITATION

As you begin to experience the benefits of daily meditation, you may want to learn more about other meditative techniques. Some forms of meditation use syllables of the Sanskrit alphabet to form *mantras,* or primordial sounds that are repeated as a way of creating heightened awareness. This method is taught by instructors at the Chopra Center for Well Being in La Jolla, California, and by other authorities. During training, a student of primordial sound meditation receives a personal mantra based on his or her particular needs. For more information on learning this technique, consult the Sources section at the end of this book.

EXERCISE

The true purpose of exercise is to invigorate and strengthen us in body, mind, and spirit. Although for many people exercise takes the form of competitive or extremely demanding physical activities, this is clearly inappropriate when addiction in any form has destabilized the mind body system. If drugs, alcohol, unhealthy eating habits, or perhaps a combination of all of these have caused you to lead a sedentary lifestyle, you'll want to begin exercising in a way that imposes no sudden or excessive requirements on your body. Conversely, if you've been obsessively pushing yourself to the limit in your work, moderate exercise will also be most beneficial.

Think of exercise as an opportunity for *understanding*. As you move your body, begin to hear and interpret the sensations that pass through your limbs. What do you learn about yourself, both physically and emotionally? If you've been subject to addiction for any length of time, you may learn that you're decidedly out of shape. You may also learn that you want to stop too soon or continue too long. These insights are as important as anything exercise will do for your muscles and tendons. They are the beginnings of reopened communication with your physical self, communication that may have long been shut down owing to the Vata imbalances brought on by addiction of any kind.

GENERAL GUIDELINES

Use the three principles below to guide you when you're beginning an exercise program. Even when you've gained more experience, they can still be very useful. They're very different from the competition-oriented "work ethic" that is often associated with exercise in the West, but they are fundamental to an Ayurvedic view of how the body can be used to enhance the spirit.

• *Exercise only to 50 percent of your capacity.* Most people worry that they haven't exerted themselves enough, but too much exertion is no better than too little. Even if you haven't exercised for a while, once you begin a physical activity you'll be able to estimate your total capacity with a good deal of accuracy. After swimming five laps, for example, you may feel that you could swim a total of twenty if you really had to—so you should stop after swimming no more than ten laps. Remember that the purpose of exercise is not to push yourself to exhaustion, but to create higher levels of energy and endurance. As your physical condition improves, your halfway-to-the-limit point will naturally increase, so following this 50 percent principle will in no way prevent you from attaining high levels of performance.

• *Try to exercise every day.* If you no longer look forward to exercise—if you feel like you're burned out after you've exercised three or four days in a row—you've probably been pushing yourself past the 50 percent limit. An exercise program must be enjoyable and self-motivating if it is to continue for any length of time. By replacing the idea of "no pain, no gain" with "no strain, maximum gain," you can gain the benefits of exercise without depleting your energy reserves.

• *Use your breathing and perspiration as measures of exercise intensity.* If you find that you have to breathe through your mouth while you're exercising, this is another indication that you're working too hard. Gasping breath and heavy perspiration mean that too much stress is being placed upon the body. Your breathing rate is one of the best indicators of exercise effectiveness. If you're breathing slowly and deeply, but without strain, you are working at the correct level.

EXERCISE AND THE DOSHAS

Ayurveda teaches that every human being is unique, and the truth of this is especially clear with regard to exercise. Just as no single prescription of a drug is best for everyone, there is no exercise program that is appropriate for every individual. However, certain principles of exercise can be applied to the three basic mind body types.

In general, Kapha types benefit from vigorous and fairly demanding exercise. With their often heavy and muscular builds, Kaphas should feel free to challenge themselves and should resist their natural tendency toward a sedentary lifestyle. Pitta types, on the other hand, tend to demand too much from their bodies. If Pitta is your dominant dosha, your orientation should be toward relaxing activities that are more recreational than competitive. For Vata types, light exercise is best—this is especially important since, as we've seen, addictive behaviors almost always produce a Vata imbalance regardless of an individual's normal doshic makeup.

Short hikes, low-stress aerobics, and light bicycling are all suitable activities for balancing Vata, but yoga exercises may be best of all. Although many people still associate yoga with strenuous postures, trances, and ascetic lifestyles, these are misconceptions. Yoga means "union" in Sanskrit, and its true purpose is to unify body, mind, and spirit. Yoga exercises certainly have benefits for the muscles and the cardiovascular system, but they also calm anxiety and focus the mind. These are qualities that make yoga especially effective in pacifying Vata.

Because Vata is associated with the elements of air and space, it is pacified by yoga postures that create a "grounding" effect by bending the body at its center or by bringing the head down toward the ground. These poses should be performed as a slow, relaxed sequence. As with any yoga exercise, it is important to remember that proper breathing is as important as the pose itself. Try to breathe deeply and rhythmically through your nose. Use your breathing to create a sense of balance, calm, and inner strength.

VATA-BALANCING POSES

As you perform these exercises, remember to relax and assume the poses without force. Don't feel you have to execute each pose perfectly. Just stretch your body to a point where you're aware of a gentle pressure. With practice, you'll naturally become more flexible.

FORWARD BEND (*PADAHASTASANA*)

Stand in a relaxed position with your arms comfortably at your sides. As you inhale, slowly raise your arms upward until they are stretched above your head. Bend your head backward until you feel a gentle stretch, and raise your eyes upward.

Keeping your elbows straight and your hands extended, bend forward at the waist and try to touch the floor in front of your toes. Stretch only as far as is comfortable, and don't feel you have to keep your knees locked. Remain bent at the waist for

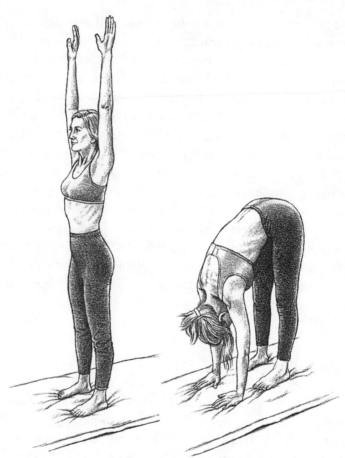

a count of five, then return to a standing posture as you inhale deeply. Repeat the exercise 3–5 times.

THUNDERBOLT POSE (*VAJRASANA*)

Kneel with your knees together and your weight resting back on your heels. Comfortably point your toes so that the soles of your feet face upward. Keep your back straight and your head up and allow your palms to rest on your knees.

Close your eyes and breathe deeply and evenly. Let your mind become clear. Maintain the pose for at least 30 seconds, or for as long as comfortable.

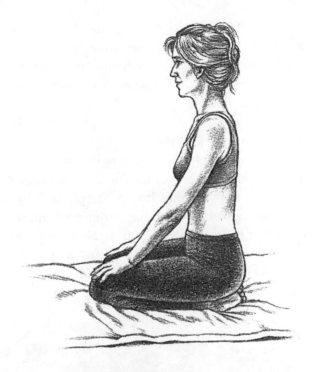

HEAD-TO-KNEE POSE (*JANU SIRSASANA*)

Sit on the floor with your legs stretched out in front of you. Bend your left knee and place the sole of your left foot flat against the inside of your right thigh. As you exhale, bend forward at the waist and reach to grasp your right foot with both hands. Don't strain, and allow yourself to bend your right

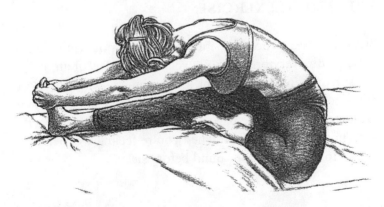

knee slightly, if necessary. Try to avoid collapsing your chest or allowing your back to become overly rounded.

Breathe normally, and hold this pose for a count of five. Then return to a sitting posture, and reverse the pose. Perform 3–5 cycles.

AWARENESS POSE (*SAVASANA*)

Lie flat on your back with your palms open, facing upward beside your legs. Close your eyes and attempt to completely relax every area of your body. Breathe deeply and rhythmically, and feel the tension disappearing from your muscles. You may practice this pose for as long as convenient—the longer the better. True relaxation is an art, and as you gain experience you'll feel yourself becoming more adept.

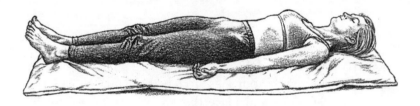

BREATHING EXERCISES

Breathing is a process of intimate connection with the universe. With every breath, you exchange billions of atoms with the surrounding environment. Nourishment is taken into the mind body system and waste is eliminated. The two exercises presented here can help you use your breathing to pacify a Vata imbalance. Use them when you're feeling worried or upset, or to help settle your mind before sleep.

ALTERNATE NOSTRIL BREATHING (NADI SHODHANA)

- Sit comfortably in a straight-backed chair with your feet flat on the floor. Place the thumb of your right hand beside your right nostril, and the two middle fingers beside your left nostril.
- Gently close the right nostril with your thumb as you slowly *exhale* through the left nostril. Now *inhale* easily through the left nostril.
- Close the left nostril with your two middle fingers and *exhale* out the right nostril. Then *inhale* easily through the right nostril.
- Once again, close the right nostril with your thumb as you slowly *exhale* through the left nostril. Now *inhale* easily through the left nostril.
- Close your left nostril with your two middle fingers and *exhale* through the right nostril. Then *inhale* easily through the right nostril.
- Over a period of 4–5 minutes, perform three complete cycles of this exercise with each nostril.

BUMBLEBEE (BHRIMARI)

- Sit in a comfortable chair with your back straight and your feet flat on the floor. *Inhale* deeply, and as you *exhale* through your nose make a low humming sound deep in your throat.
- When your breath is exhausted, *inhale* again and repeat the humming sound as you *exhale*.
- Perform five cycles of this exercise over a period of 2–3 minutes.

12

VATA-BALANCING DIET

In the early stages of recovery from addictive behaviors, a diet that balances Vata dosha is especially important. The recommendations that follow are designed for this purpose.

1. *Favor* foods that are warm, heavy, and oily. *Minimize* foods that are cold, dry, and light.
2. *Favor* foods that are sweet, sour, and salty. *Minimize* foods that are spicy, bitter, and astringent.
3. Eat larger quantities, but not more than you can digest easily.

SOME SPECIFIC RECOMMENDATIONS

- **Dairy.** All dairy products pacify Vata.
- **Sweeteners.** All sweeteners are good (in moderation) for pacifying Vata.
- **Oils.** All oils reduce Vata.

- **Grains.** Rice and wheat are very good. *Reduce* barley, corn, millet, buckwheat, rye, and oats.
- **Fruits.** *Favor* sweet, sour, or heavy fruits, such as oranges, bananas, avocados, grapes, cherries, peaches, melons, berries, plums, pineapples, mangoes, and papayas. *Reduce* dry or light fruits, such as apples, pears, pomegranates, cranberries, and dried fruits.
- **Vegetables.** Beets, cucumbers, carrots, asparagus, and sweet potatoes are good. They should be cooked, not raw. The following vegetables are acceptable in moderate quantities if they're cooked, especially with ghee or oil and Vata-reducing spices: peas, broccoli, cauliflower, celery, zucchini, and green leafy vegetables. It's better to avoid sprouts and cabbage.
- **Spices.** Cardamom, cumin, ginger, cinnamon, salt, cloves, mustard seed, and small quantities of black pepper are good.
- **Nuts.** All nuts are good.
- **Beans.** *Reduce* all beans, *except* tofu and split mung-bean soup.
- **Meat and fish** (for nonvegetarians). Chicken, turkey, and seafoods are all right. Beef should be avoided.

13

JOY—THE REAL ANSWER

It would seem that the psychology and biology of addictive behaviors have been investigated from every possible angle. Much of this work has been very valuable—yet the phenomenon of addiction in all its forms is still with us, and is even growing in many segments of the population. I am certainly not the first to suggest that a spiritually based approach, together with up-to-date scientific information, offers the best opportunity for dealing successfully with addiction. I've already mentioned my respect for the twelve-step programs created by Alcoholics Anonymous and other organizations, and now, in closing, I'd like to offer my own twelve points for replacing addictive behavior with true joy in living.

In Part One, I made a distinction between happiness and joy. I described happiness as a feeling that is triggered by an external experience, such as finding some money on the ground, while joy originates essentially from within. Joy is a return to the deep harmony of body, mind, and spirit that was yours at birth and that can be yours again. Once this has been recaptured, there is no need for stimulants, depressants, or anything else that must be bought, hidden, injected, inhaled, turned on, or turned off. You needed none of these things in childhood, when a sunny day and the love of your family was enough to fill you with joy. That openness to love, that capacity for wholeness with the world around you, is still within you. If addiction has been a part of your life for some time, you may feel it is impossible to regain your pre-addicted self. But it *is* possible. In fact, it's inevitable, when you let go of guilt and recrimination and begin to bring joyful experiences into your life. The suggestions below are intended to help you do that.

Because I don't want these suggestions to seem in any way like a list of commandments etched in stone, I've put them in the form of questions. Please note that none of these questions says anything about addiction, nor is there any mention of abstinence or avoidance. These are simply things you can do to open yourself to health, to joy, and indeed to life itself.

I urge you to read over this list from time to time, ideally at the end of a day. If you've been able to experience one of these activities, how did it make you feel? If you were unable to do so today, is there some way you can find an opportunity tomorrow?

1. *Did you get the right amount of sleep last night?* Some people need more sleep than others, and the number of hours that's best for you depends on your age, your mind body type, and many other factors. But research has shown that both excessive sleep and insomnia are signs of depression—and many addicted people, of course, are quite understandably depressed. If you're sleeping more than ten hours a night, or less than six, this is probably an area in which you can make some positive adjustments. For more information on sleep and its benefits, you may want to consult my book *Restful Sleep,* which is also part of the Perfect Health Library series.

2. *Did you start your day with nurturing activities that*

strengthened you in body and in spirit? The first hours are crucial in determining your state of mind throughout the day. If possible, try to wake up without using an alarm clock, but if you do need an alarm, use a clock radio tuned to soothing music. Don't feel you have to listen to the news or turn on the television first thing in the morning. Very often these provide negative information that can start you off on the wrong foot. As for breakfast, Ayurveda teaches that if taken at all it should be a light meal, but if you truly enjoy a big breakfast it's better to eat one than to start the day with stressful avoidance. The early morning, of course, is an ideal time to meditate, and as this becomes part of your life you'll naturally begin to prefer lighter morning meals.

3. *Did you find real pleasure in your work?* Lack of fulfillment at work is one of the most frequently cited causes of the depression that gives rise to addictive behavior. If you find your work unrewarding, any financial benefits you may be receiving can hardly compensate for the damage that's being done to your overall enjoyment of life. It's been said that a genius is someone who is able to invent his or her own occupation, and there's no doubt that work should be an opportunity for creativity and growth. Even if you can't make radical career changes at this point, look for areas outside your present job that you may be able to develop over time. I'm glad that I was able to accomplish this with my writing, although for many years I also had a full-time medical practice.

4. *If you felt angry at someone or something, were you able to express this in a constructive way?* It's often harmful to express anger suddenly and emotionally, but it's also a mistake to simply hold it in and let the destructive feelings fester within yourself. According to Ayurveda, anger should be "digested" just like anything else that's taken into the body. A key factor in this process is recognizing that anger is created by you, not by anything someone else says or does. No matter what happens, the choice of how to respond is always yours. Once you

learn how to exercise this choice, you'll have the ability to thoroughly process anger just as your body processes food and drink. When this emotional digestion has taken place, you can then express your feelings to others without harm to yourself or to them.

5. *Were you able to experience nature today with awareness and appreciation?* Ayurveda teaches that there is a universal life force, called *prana* in Sanskrit, from which all living things draw energy. Healthy food is one source of prana, but food is by no means the only source or even the most important. Even if you live and work in an urban area, you can keep in touch with nature through contact with plants and flowers, by walking in a park or near a body of water whenever there's time, or even simply by being out in the sunlight for a while each day. Just by planting a seed in a flowerpot, for example, diligently watering it, and lovingly observing the growth of a flower, you can have a genuinely rich experience of nature. The level of mindfulness and awareness that you bring to such prana-enhancing activities is actually much more significant than the activities themselves.

6. *Did you find time for enjoyable activities or exercise?* Over the last twenty years, a substantial body of research has demonstrated that a category of hormones known as endorphins can have highly beneficial effects both physically and emotionally. Exercise is one of the most effective ways of stimulating the brain to produce endorphins, and this accounts for the "runner's high" familiar to many athletes. But you don't have to engage in strenuous activities to gain these benefits. The yoga poses described in chapter 11 are designed to ignite the body's energy centers, which Ayurveda calls *marma* points. These points are the bases for stimulating energy from within. Moreover, yoga requires neither the time nor the financial investment that other forms of exercise demand. Even if you can devote only a few minutes each day to it, yoga can provide many of the benefits of meditation while strengthening your

body at the same time. Your improved physical condition will make you much less inclined toward self-destructive activities.

7. *Were you able to spend some quiet time by yourself?* The presence of "static" in many forms is characteristic of modern life, and it can be extremely anxiety-provoking. The ability to enter and enjoy silence is the antidote to static, and gaining access to the silent spaces between your thoughts is the real purpose of Ayurvedic meditation. The small amount of self-discipline that meditation requires will be more than repaid by the rich experience of restful alertness, which is paradoxically both quieting and stimulating at the same time. I am convinced that meditation is the single most effective technique for ending addiction in any form.

8. *Did you laugh with real pleasure today?* There are many kinds of laughter, just as there are many kinds of speech. As a result of stress or anger, many people forget how to laugh with real happiness, and a great deal of today's humor is based on put-downs or watching someone else's misfortunes. Heartless laughter can be very destructive, but laughter that is filled with warmth and joy is almost magical in its ability to heal both physical and emotional pain. Try remembering some things that have really made you laugh heartily at one time or another; you might even enjoy writing them down. What, for instance, are the three most genuinely funny incidents you've ever seen? These are moments to treasure, and you should allow yourself to think of them whenever you feel overwhelmed by negative feelings. Laughter can truly be a positive addiction, and its presence can overshadow the impulse toward other addictive behaviors.

9. *If you felt tired or under stress, were you able to rest for a while?* Most people feel as if they never have enough time, but of course no one has any more time than anyone else. When dealing with the Vata imbalance that is commonly caused by addiction, you must honor the need for rest in the midst of what may seem like impossible situations. Ayurveda

teaches that certain periods of the day are naturally suited for relaxation. These periods are dominated by Kapha, the calmest and most stable of the doshas, and they occur between six and ten o'clock, in both the morning and the evening. If possible, use these times as quiet, unhurried segments of the day. The Kapha periods are ideal for meditation, but even after meditating it is enormously beneficial to remain at ease during these blocks of time in the morning and evening. The world won't collapse if you simply take it easy for a while. In fact, it will seem to run much more smoothly during the rest of your day.

10. *Did you take your meals in pleasant surroundings, with company you enjoyed?* According to Ayurveda, the food that comprises a meal is less significant than the emotions that accompany it. Even the emotions of the people who created the meal are very important. Although we've grown accustomed to the idea of "fast food" and all that it implies, a capacity for real enjoyment of food is absolutely central to a genuine enjoyment of life. And until you're able to genuinely enjoy life, addiction and other self-destructive behaviors may continue to be a problem. Try to make at least one meal a day a truly pleasant and leisurely occasion. If possible, Ayurveda recommends making it the midday meal.

11. *Did you show love today to friends and family members?* Love can be shown in many ways. Human beings best perceive affection through the sense of touch, and physical contact is clearly a wonderful way of expressing love. Talking, listening, sharing a meal, taking a walk together in the evening, listening to music with people you care for are also among the many ways of showing affection, yet it's so easy to lose sight of them under the pressures of contemporary life. You can't schedule affection the way you can set aside times for meditation or exercise, but you can be mindfully aware of your love for the people close to you, and you can find a way to express those feelings at any time, spontaneously and joyfully. In all of life there is nothing more healthy or important.

12. *Did you freely and joyfully receive their love in return?* Once you realize that you are loved by many people—that your very existence is a manifestation of love—you will be free of the need for addiction. Love is the greatest treasure. Compared to love, no addictive substance has any power whatsoever.

The topics we have considered in this book are only a very few of the most common addictions found in modern America. There are also people who are addicted to shopping, to debt, to driving over the speed limit, to collecting, and to hundreds of other behaviors. Certain people are even addicted to surgery. It's been said that we live in a society of addiction— that we're addicted to addiction—and perhaps there's truth in this. To the extent that addiction represents a search for fulfillment in areas where real fulfillment can never be found, I do think that addiction is a defining characteristic of contemporary life. However, I also believe that our determinedly materialistic orientation is now beginning to evolve toward a real recognition of spiritual values. This change, more than any adjustment in laws or penalties, represents the best hope for reducing or eliminating the problem of addiction. If your life has been damaged by addictive behavior, the very fact that you are reading this book suggests that you are participating in the important shift in perspective that's now taking place, away from the illusory pleasures of substances and stimulants, and toward the inner joy—the genuine *ecstasy*—that is to be found in your spiritual self.

Starting right now, be proud of your sincere intention, and begin to enjoy the truly infinite possibilities that every moment of your life holds forth.

BIBLIOGRAPHY

Chopra, Deepak. *Unconditional Life: Mastering the Forces That Shape Personal Reality*. New York: Bantam Books, 1991.

———. *Perfect Health*. New York: Harmony Books, 1991.

Condry, John C. *The Psychology of Television*. Hillsdale, N.J.: L. Erlbaum Associates, 1989.

Diagnostic and Statistical Manual of Mental Disorders, Fourth Edition. Washington, D.C.: American Psychiatric Association, 1994.

Doweiko, Harold E. *Concepts of Chemical Dependency*. Pacific Grove, Calif.: Brooks/Cole Publishing Company, 1996.

Frawley, David, O.M.D. *Ayurvedic Healing: A Comprehensive Guide*. Salt Lake City: Passage Press, 1989.

Gelernter, David. *1939: The Lost World of the Fair*. New York: Avon Books, 1995.

Johnson, Robert A. *Ecstasy: Understanding the Psychology of Joy.* San Francisco: HarperCollins, 1987.

Ludwig, Arnold M., M.D. *Understanding the Alcoholic's Mind.* New York: Oxford University Press, 1988.

Milkman, Harvey, and Sunderwerth, Stanley. *Craving for Ecstasy: The Consciousness and Chemistry of Escape.* New York: Lexington Books, 1987.

Phillips, Adam. *On Kissing, Tickling and Being Bored: Psychoanalytic Essays on the Unexamined Life.* Cambridge: Harvard University Press, 1993.

Regis, Edward. *Who Got Einstein's Office?: Eccentricity and Genius at the Institute for Advanced Study.* Reading, Mass.: Addison-Wesley, 1987.

Szasz, Thomas. *Ceremonial Chemistry.* Garden City, N.Y.: Anchor/Doubleday, 1974.

Weil, Andrew, and Rosen, Winifred. *From Chocolate to Morphine: Everything You Need to Know About Mind-Altering Drugs.* Boston: Houghton Mifflin, 1983.

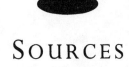

SOURCES

More information on Mind Body and Ayurvedic treatments, products, herbs, and educational programs can be obtained from the following organizations:

Infinite Possibilities International
P.O. Box 1088
Sudbury, MA 01776
(800) 858-1808 or (508) 440-8400

The Chopra Center for Well Being
7630 Fay Avenue
La Jolla, CA 92037
(888) 4-CHOPRA or (619) 551-7788

Ayurvedic Institute
1311 Menaul N.E., Suite A
Albuquerque, NM 87112
(505) 291-9698

American Institute of Vedic Studies
P.O. Box 8357
Sante Fe, NM 87504

American School of Ayurvedic Science
10025 N.E. 4th Street
Bellevue, WA 98004

Maharishi Ayurved Products
Colorado Springs, CO
(800) 255-8332

Deepak Chopra and Infinite Possibilities International offer a
wide range of seminars, products, and educational programs.
For additional information, please contact: Infinite Possibilities
International, 60 Union Avenue, Sudbury, MA 01776, U.S.A.
1-800-858-1808 (toll-free) / (508) 440-8400. For medical in-
quiries and health-related programs, please contact: The Chopra
Center for Well Being, 7630 Fay Avenue, La Jolla, CA 92037,
U.S.A. 1-888-424-6772 (toll-free) / (619) 551-7788.

INDEX

ABOUT THE AUTHOR

Deepak Chopra, M.D., is the author of more than fifty books translated in over thirty-five languages, including numerous *New York Times* bestsellers in both the fiction and non fiction categories. Chopra's Wellness Radio airs weekly on Sirius Stars, Channel 102 which focuses on the areas of success, love, sexuality and relationships, well being, and spirituality. He is founder and president of the Alliance for a New Humanity. *Time* magazine heralds Deepak Chopra as one of the top 100 heroes and icons of the century, and credits him as "the poet-prophet of alternative medicine."

www.deepakchopra.com